HEALTH FROM NATURE

Vitamins & Minerals : *Their role in the body, daily requirement, natural sources, food supplements and toxicity.*

Herbal Remedies : *The endless potential of herbs and plants.*

Aromatherapy : *Sweet-smelling oils and plant extracts for healing.*

Bach Flowers : *Solutions to "body-mind" treatment problems in plants.*

HEALTH *from* NATURE

The Ultimate Guide to Physical and Mental Well-being

JON TILLMAN • DAN WOLF
KEVIN HUDSON • SUSAN HOLDEN

New Age Books

ISBN: 81-7822-246-9

First Indian Edition: Delhi, 2005

(First published 2003, by Astrolog Publishing House, Israel.)

Published by
NEW AGE BOOKS
A-44 Naraina Phase-I
New Delhi-110 028 (INDIA)
Email: nab@vsnl.in
Website: www.newagebooksindia.com

For Sale in Indian Subcontinent Only

Printed in India
at Shri Jainendra Press
A-45 Naraina Phase-I, New Delhi-110 028

This publication contains the opinions and ideas of its authors. It is intended to provide helpful and informative material on the subject matter covered. It is sold with the understanding that the authors and publisher are not engaged in rendering professional services in the book. If the reader requires personal assistance or advice, a competent professional should be consulted.

The authors, book producer, and publisher specifically disclaim any responsibility for any liability, loss or risk, personal or otherwise, which is incurred as a consequence, directly or indirectly, of the use and application of any of the contents of this book.

Jon Tillman

Vitamins

Introduction

The word vitamin comes from the Latin word vita, meaning "life," and the word amine, which is a derivative of ammonia. The name was coined by the biochemist, Casimir Funk, in 1911.

The dictionary definition of the word vitamin is: "any of a group of organic substances essential in small quantities to normal metabolism, found in minute amounts in natural foodstuffs and also produced synthetically."

One of the strangest things about vitamins is that until almost 90 years ago, no one even knew that they existed. You may ask, "If man survived for millennia without knowing about vitamins, what is all the fuss about today?"

Well, I'll give you three reasons.

Wherever people lived in the world, they suffered from diseases such as beriberi, pellagra, scurvy, rickets, and so on. Scientists understood that the cause of these diseases was a missing factor in their diets.

As the global population grew, and agricultural land decreased, chemical fertilizers were used to augment food production (as well as the profits of farmers and manufacturers of processed foods). Processed foods and foods that are grown on chemically fertilized land do not contain the amount of vitamins and minerals necessary for the ongoing, normal functioning of the body.

Healing by means of vitamins has become accepted practice. However, the optimal conditions for enjoying a healthy life - proper nutrition containing all the required nutrients, pure water, fresh air, sufficient exercise, and sufficient rest - are almost impossible to achieve in our rushed, tense, polluted lifestyles.

In this book, I will try to explain what the lack of these factors causes, and why there is a lack - basing my arguments on the school of thought that claims that the lacks that are caused by our lifestyle and the tensions surrounding us must be supplemented with natural food supplements.

Some people think that if we eat correctly - vegetables, fruit, dairy products, grains, legumes and meats - there can be no shortage of vitamins and minerals. Research has shown that this is simply not true - that entire segments of the population suffer from a lack of vitamins and minerals. This is a major cause of the diseases that are prevalent in this day and age. It's impossible, for example, to escape cigarette smoke, exhaust or industrial fumes, and pesticides (even if we eat organically grown fruit and vegetables). These are major factors in insufficient vitamin consumption. The way to get around this problem is by natural food supplements.

This book presents the foodstuffs that contain the components or the supplements that we need, but it is not a substitute for consulting naturopaths, homeopaths, physicians, or dieticians who specialize in natural food supplements and components. Of course, there are differences between groups of people - men and women, children and adults, adolescent girls and pregnant women -

as well as between individuals. However, there are some basic rules of correct nutrition.

Certain misconceptions exist. For example, some people think that vitamins are energy pills, or food substitutes. They think that by taking vitamins, they don't have to eat "real food." This is absolutely incorrect. In fact, vitamins cannot be absorbed or assimilated by the digestive system without food. I hope to clarify these erroneous beliefs in this book.

Vitamins per se do not contain calories, and they are certainly not substitutes for protein or any other nutrient, such as starches, minerals, fats, and so on. Vitamins themselves are not part of the components of our bodies, and there is no way at all, even in theory, that we can take vitamins instead of eating food, and be healthy.

How do vitamins operate? Well, you could compare them to the spark plugs in a car. Vitamins regulate the process of metabolism in the body by means of the enzymatic systems; they are part of the requisite components of these systems, regulating the tasks and functions of the body.

Compared to the required amounts of other components such as proteins, fats and carbohydrates, the required amounts of vitamins (even in megadoses) are minuscule, and are measured in milligrams (mg) or even in micrograms (mcg). Having said that, a lack of even one (!) vitamin is liable to jeopardize the whole system.

There are six types of nutrients: vitamins, minerals, carbohydrates, fats, proteins, and water, and they are absorbed into the body via the digestive system and into the bloodstream. Vitamins are produced in nature. However, synthetic vitamins are produced in laboratories. Although their chemical formula may be identical to that of natural vitamins, the difference between them is like day and night. It is always preferable to use the natural form of vitamins.

Vitamins are divided into two groups: oil-soluble vitamins and water-soluble vitamins. Natural, oil-soluble vitamins (A, D, E, and K) are found in oils. They are absorbed from the intestine together with the fats.(lipids) from food, so that if the absorption of fats in the intestine is impaired, or if there is a shortage of fats, the absorption of the vitamins will also be impaired. The use of bad oil (such as mineral oil) is also counter-productive. Oil-soluble vitamins are not excreted during urination, and are stored in the liver. They are heat-stable, and are not destroyed as easily during food processing as water-soluble vitamins.

Water-soluble vitamins (B complex and C) are not stored in the body, as they are excreted during urination. This means that they must be taken on a daily basis. They are more easily absorbed than oil-soluble vitamins, and are very important in the metabolism of fats and proteins.

Vitamins

Vitamin A

Although vitamin A was officially identified only in 1931, its connection with sight and night-blindness has been known for centuries. Millennia ago, the ancient Egyptians were aware that eating liver combated night-blindness.

Vitamin A, like D, E and K, belongs to the category of oil-soluble vitamins. It is also an anti-oxidant (that is, it does not combine with oxygen), as are vitamins C and E. While vitamin A is found only in natural products, such as cod-liver oil, the human body is able to convert carotene into vitamin A in the liver and the walls of the intestines.

Carotene comes in several forms: Alpha and gamma-carotene are found in green leafy vegetables. One molecule of vitamin A is produced from one molecule of alpha or gamma-carotene. Beta-carotene is found in orange fruit and vegetables, and one molecule of vitamin A is produced from two molecules of beta-carotene.

Vitamins are interdependent: this means that they need each other in order to prevent rapid breakdown, to enhance absorption, and so on. Vitamin E prevents the rapid breakdown of vitamin A, so it should be consumed in conjunction with vitamin A. Vitamin A protects vitamin C from oxidation. Zinc extracts vitamin A from the liver, where it is stored. Vitamin A interacts well with calcium, zinc, phosphorus, as well as vitamins B (complex), D, and E.

Vitamin A plays a vital role in protecting epithelial tissues; these include the coverings of inner tissues, membranes, gland sacs, and their drainage system. Vitamin A also protects the outer coverings of the teeth and gums. It reinforces immunity to respiratory infections, accelerates recovery from diseases, and stimulates blood coagulation. It strengthens hair and bones, and helps get rid of liver-spots (that form as a result of aging). Other skin ailments such as acne benefit from vitamin A. Vitamin A is effective in treating hyperthyroidism, and, in its beta-carotene form, certain cases of cancer. People who take cholesterol-reducing medication, as well as women who are on the contraceptive pill, need vitamin A.

The average recommended daily amount of vitamin A for children is 2,100 IU (international units) daily for infants and children up to one year, 2,000 IU for children up to three years, 2,500 for children up to six years, and 4,000-5,000 IU for youngsters up to 18 years. For adults, it is 4,000-6,000 IU. This can vary, according to individual needs.

Vitamin A can be found in the following foods: fish, especially the liver, butter, cream cheese, and egg-yolks. Carotene is present in vegetables such as spinach, cabbage, parsley, scallions, chives, green peas, chickpeas, corn, okra, fresh lentils, cumin seeds, carrots, yams, pumpkin, beets, red peppers, and malva. It is found in fruits such as apricots, mangos, persimmons, orange guavas, melons, peaches, tomatoes, and papaya. It is also contained in almonds, filberts, wheat-germ oil, whole-wheat flour, and soybeans.

How can we identify a lack of vitamin A? The symptoms include xerophthalmia (no secretion of tears from the tear-ducts), swollen eyelids, night-blindness or even difficulty in seeing in dim light, susceptibility to chills and respiratory, urinary, and sinus infections. The skin may become rough, dry, and scaly, and there could be outbreaks of acne and white spots. The reproductive system can be problematic, resulting in miscarriages or abnormal fetal development.

Before we go on a spinach or cod-liver oil binge, it is important to know that excessive consumption of vitamin A has toxic side-effects, resulting in nausea, vomiting, diarrhea, hair loss, skin and vision problems, irregular periods, headaches, and an enlarged liver. The safest thing is to take natural vitamin A - in the form of beta-carotene - which has no toxicity. At worst, overdosing will cause the skin to take on a yellowish tinge.

The Vitamin B Group

Water-soluble vitamin B1 is also called thiamine, and it is responsible for the metabolism of carbohydrates (starches). If there is a lack of vitamin B1, it can lead to a malfunctioning of the nerves. In extreme cases, it can result in beriberi, a disease of the nerves which culminates in paralysis and congestive heart failure. The link between deficient vitamin B1 and beriberi was identified in 1642. The presence of vitamin B1 permits the secretion of the neurotransmitter, acetylcholine, when transmitting stimuli to the central nervous system and to the muscles. This action is inhibited when vitamin B1 is lacking.

Vitamin B1 is essential for growth. This means that it is very important to give children healthful, unprocessed foods, such as whole-wheat flour (instead of processed white flour), brown rice (instead of white rice), and other whole grains. A diet that consists entirely of processed foodstuffs, without any supplementary vitamin B1, will lead to stunted growth as well as defective action of the heart muscle.

Vitamin B1

Vitamin B1 is easily destroyed by alcohol, smoking, and chemicals in foods and medications; it is therefore given in large doses in order to strengthen the immune system, and to combat problems of alcohol consumption and smoking, and to women who are either on the Pill or are pregnant.

Vitamin B1 and the other B-complex vitamins are interdependent, and it is especially important to take vitamins B2 and B6 in conjunction with B1.

Vitamin B1 improves the appetite and enhances growth. It helps convert carbohydrates into glucose (sugar), and is beneficial for digestion, especially of carbohydrates. It protects the nervous system, and improves the mental condition. It is useful in the treatment of shingles and toothache, and combats motion sickness and seasickness.

The recommended average daily dose of vitamin B1 for children up to one year is 0.3-0.5 mg, for children up to six is 0.9 mg, for children up to 10 is 1.2 mg, and for youngsters up to 18 is 1.1-1.4 mg. For adults, it is 1.4-1.6 mg. This can vary, according to individual needs, as mentioned before.

Vitamin B1 can be found in the following foodstuffs: brewer's yeast, sunflower seeds, peanuts, corn, bran, brown rice, wheat-germ, whole sesame seeds, brazil nuts, alfalfa tablets, pine nuts, whole-wheat flour, soy flour, oats, fresh vegetables, lentils, and most fruits.

A vitamin B1 deficiency, as we mentioned before, can lead to beriberi - which is muscle debilitation and dystrophy - as well as a pounding heartbeat (although here caution must be exercised: the condition could be the result of something else), excessive pressure in the veins, and damage to the heart muscle. It can also cause the loss of knee and ankle reflexes, fatigue, loss of appetite, and digestive problems. Mental confusion, forgetfulness, fears, and a lack of stability are other possible results of a lack of vitamin B1.

It is not possible to overdose on vitamin B1, since it is water-soluble, and the surplus is expelled in the urine. However, a massive dose can occasionally cause palpitations, tremors, and allergies.

Vitamin B2

Vitamin B2, which is also known as riboflavin, is sometimes called vitamin G. It was identified in 1926, and isolated in 1932. Vitamin B2 is a key factor in many physical processes, such as conveying hydrogen, and converting carbo-hydrates and amino acids into fatty acids; it is also linked to the production of enzymes and coenzymes. Like vitamin A, it plays an important role in vision. It is linked to oxidation in the body's tissues, and mainly in the binding of hydrogen and oxygen. The need for vitamin B2 varies in accordance with the rate of protein absorption.

While regular cooking does not destroy it, it disappears in water, and, as it is extremely photosensitive - especially to UV - in light.

As we mentioned above, vitamin B2 assists in the metabolism of proteins, fats and carbohydrates, and for this reason, is particularly important for people who eat red meat. It is important for the conversion of the essential amino acid, tryptophan, to niacin. In addition, vitamin B2 helps the eyes to adjust to light, and safeguards the health of the skin, especially the lips, tongue, and corners of the mouth. It is vital for growth, and the reproductive system, as well as for women who take the Pill or are pregnant. Diabetics and ulcer-sufferers also need vitamin B2.

The recommended average daily dose for children up to the age of one year is up to 0.4-0.6 mg, for children up to six years is up to 1 mg, and for youngsters up to 18 years is 1.3-1.6 mg. For adults, it ranges between 1.2 and 1.3 mg, but the amount can be increased in cases of pregnancy, the Pill, diabetes, stress and red-meat consumption.

Vitamin B2 can be found in the following foodstuffs: brewer's yeast and torula yeast, avocado, parsley, coriander, broccoli, okra, artichokes, yams, garlic, corn, fresh mushrooms, most vegetables and fruits, seaweed, egg yolks, fish, milk, cheese, whole-wheat bread, whole sesame, almonds, brazil nuts and walnuts, lentils, and buckwheat.

A vitamin B2 deficiency can be recognized by symptoms such as sores and fissures at the corners of the mouth, or a red, shiny tongue. Another indication is redness in the whites of the eyes, as well as soreness and fatigue in the eyes. Eye problems could even include blindness and cataracts. There could be a deficiency in the production of red blood cells, causing anemia. Greasy skin, eczema, dizziness, difficulty in urinating, and vaginal itching are other symptoms of vitamin B2 deficiency.

How toxic can vitamin B2 be? Not at all, as it is a water-soluble vitamin, and any surplus is excreted in the urine. However, excessive amounts of vitamin B2 could cause itching and numbness in the limbs.

Just to reassure you: Vitamin B2 tends to dye the urine a bright yellow. Don't let this alarm you.

Vitamin B3

Vitamin B3 is known by several names: nicotinic acid (niacinamide), nicotinamide, or the anti-pellagra (rough skin) vitamin. If there are sufficient amounts of vitamins B1, B2 and B6, 60 mg of the amino acid tryptophan will produce 1 mg of B3.

Vitamin B3 is absorbed in the small intestine, and stored in the liver. Its principal function is the production of important coenzymes for the oxidation of the tissues. It helps enzymes which break down proteins, fat and carbohydrates.

Another of its vital functions is the production of sex hormones - estrogen, progesterone, testosterone - as well as of cortisone, thyroxin, and insulin. It is important for the functioning of the brain and nervous system.

While this vitamin is not sensitive to air, light or heat, it is destroyed when cooked in water, or by alcohol; this explains why alcoholics suffer from a serious lack of vitamin B3. Women who take the Pill (which contains estrogen) also need a B3 supplement, since estrogen destroys this vitamin. Antibiotics also destroy B3, as does sulfa.

As we can see, vitamin B3 is very important for our bodies. However, it has many other functions:

It improves blood circulation and lowers high blood pressure; it helps lower a high cholesterol level, it fortifies the digestive system, improves bad breath, and alleviates diarrhea; it helps with migraines, vertigo, epilepsy, and situations of mental stress, depression, or schizophrenia; it is helpful with pellagra, and makes the skin look healthier; in heart attacks, niacin reduces death by 11%; it prevents baldness and dental caries; finally, in chemotherapy, the niacinamide is responsible for expelling the destroyed cells, and reducing the damage to the DNA in the healthy ones.

In large doses, niacin can cause flushing, fever, and redness in the face and hands - so sometimes niacinamide is used instead, as it does not have these side effects. Some conditions, such as migraine, however, require niacin - and it is then taken together with equal quantities of inositol (which also belongs to the vitamin B complex). The dosage should be increased gradually.

The recommended average daily amount for children up to four years is 6-9 mg (this is the optimal dose), for children up to ten years is 16 mg, and for youngsters up to 18 is 15-18 mg. For adults, it is 12-18 mg. In natural vitamin B complex tablets, there is a sufficient amount of vitamin B3, unless conditions such as cholesterol, sun-sensitive skin or antibiotics are present, in which case the amount should be increased.

What are the sources of vitamin B3? Liver, white chicken meat, fish, eggs, most vegetables, potatoes, kelp, avocados, pumpkin, mushrooms, lentils, okra, figs, dates, wheat-germ, whole-wheat flour, buckwheat, cornstarch, brewer's yeast, roasted peanuts, pine nuts, sunflower seeds, almonds, sesame seeds, chestnuts, and pistachios.

A lack of vitamin B3 can be expressed in the following phenomena: defective production of sex hormones, cortisone, thyroxin, and insulin; digestive problems such as indigestion, heartburn, diarrhea, nausea, and a loss of appetite; memory loss (resulting from excessive consumption of corn products); "burning" limbs; weakness in the muscles; pellagra; skin infections; negative personality changes; schizophrenia; impaired learning ability and behavioral problems in children.

None of the vitamin B3 forms is toxic. The possible side effects of large doses of niacin were discussed above (over 75 mg in children, and over 100 mg in adults). However, if it is necessary to give children large amounts, their skin may take on a yellowish tinge, and they may feel a bit strange. Pets also need vitamin B3.

Vitamin B5

Vitamin B5, which is also known as pantothenic acid, calcium pantothenate or pantonol, is a vital component of every living plant or animal cell. Research on this vitamin was conducted at the beginning of the 20th century. While good nutrition supplies the necessary amount of vitamin B5, there are factors in modern foods that destroy or neutralize it.

While vitamin B5 is essential for the development of the central nervous system, and for the creation of coenzyme A, which is linked to the metabolism of carbohydrates, proteins, and fats, its most important function is the synthesis of the neurotransmitter, acetylcholine.

Pantothenic acid is required for the efficient functioning of the adrenal glands; moreover, it produces natural cortisone - and as such is an important factor in the immune system.

In order to ensure the optimal functioning of the other B complex vitamins, vitamin B5 is required. It can be produced by the bacteria in healthy intestines in both adults and children. Vitamin B5 is destroyed by heat, freezing, preservatives, and food processing, as well as by drugs containing estrogen and sulfa.

Vitamin B5 has additional functions: It assists in converting sugars and fats to energy; it is beneficial in various allergic conditions - especially in conjunction with vitamin A; it is necessary for the health of the digestive system; in high doses, it is helpful in inflammation of the joints; by creating antibodies, it is useful in cases of arthritis and other inflammatory conditions; it helps heal sores and herpes (with vitamin C); it is helpful after surgery, and helps combat toxicity resulting from antibiotics; it helps fight fatigue and stress.

The recommended average daily amount for children up to one year is 2-3 mg, for children up to three years is 3 mg, for children between four and ten years, 3-5 mg, and for youngsters up to 18 years, 4-7 mg. For adults, it ranges between 4 and 7 mg, although larger amounts can be taken in certain cases.

Where can natural vitamin B5 be found? The following foods contain it: most vegetables and fruits, green vegetables, milk, yogurt, eggs, wheat-germ, brewer's yeast, cornstarch, buckwheat, dry legumes, sunflower seeds, whole grains such as brown rice and whole-wheat flour, nuts, and inner organs, such as liver and kidneys.

If there is a shortage of vitamin B5, the following symptoms may occur: Digestive problems in the stomach, constipation, and duodenal ulcers; arthritis and inflammation of the joints; hypoglycemia; a weak immune system; skin diseases; circulatory problems, and pins and needles in the limbs; fatigue, headaches, rapid heartbeat during exertion, slack posture, and vertigo. Moreover, a lack of vitamin B5 during pregnancy could lead to birth defects.

Like the rest of members of the vitamin B complex, B5 is water-soluble, and any surplus is excreted in the urine. This means that it is not in the least toxic, even in children.

Vitamin B6

Vitamin B6, which is also known as pyridoxine, was isolated in 1938, and produced synthetically in the same year. Only in 1954, however, when a link between sterilized, synthetic baby food and convulsions and epilepsy in infants was discovered, was the importance of this vitamin understood. It transpires that the sterilization process destroys vitamin B6. The vitamin is water-soluble, like the rest of the members of the vitamin B complex, which means that it is excreted in the urine within eight hours of being consumed, and should be replenished regularly.

Vitamin B6 actually consists of pyridoxine and pyridoxinal, which are necessary for metabolism in a protein-rich diet. It plays a significant role in metabolizing carbohydrates and fats, as well. It is important for the absorption of vitamin B12, and for the production of red blood cells and stomach acids. A certain amount of it can be produced by the bacteria in the intestines.

In its pure form, vitamin B6 is heat resistant, but is sensitive to light and to heating, when this is part of processing food. It is important during pregnancy and breast-feeding, and when there is a need for magnesium. It is very useful in sickle cell anemia, edemas, and problems of dialysis in the kidneys, and is essential for people who suffer from stress, people who cannot remember their dreams, and women who take the Pill.

It has been shown that people who suffer from low levels of B6 also have sugar problems such as diabetes or hypoglycemia, and for this reason, foods in which the B6 has been destroyed by processes such as in roasting, pickling, long-term storage, and alcohol preservation, should be avoided. Vitamin B6 can reduce the amount of insulin intake in diabetes.

Among other things, vitamin B6 helps maintain the balance between sodium and potassium; it is a natural diuretic; it enables stored glycogen to be converted into glucose; it helps in the production of hydrochloric acid; it is useful with allergy problems and inflammations (of the urinary tract and joints); it helps with cramps and pains in the legs; it helps prevent skin problems, acne, and nervous problems; it helps prevent nausea (such as morning sickness, travel sickness and seasickness).

The required amount of vitamin B6 depends on how rich in protein the person's diet is: the more protein consumed, the greater the amount of B6 required. The recommended daily average amount of B6 for children up to six months old is at least 0.3 mg, for children up to three years, 0.6-0.9 mg, for children up to six years, up to 1.3 mg, for children up to 10 years, up to 1.8 mg, and for youngsters up to 18 years, 2-2.2 mg. For adults, it ranges between 2 and 2.6 mg, depending on factors such as smoking, consumption of alcohol, pregnancy, the Pill, and so on. For optimal performance of B6 in the body, equal amounts of vitamins B1, B2, C and magnesium should also be taken.

Where do we find vitamin B6? The following foods provide the body with vitamin B6: wheat germ, brewer's yeast, bran, inner organs, eggs, milk, molasses, sunflower seeds, walnuts, dried fruit, most vegetables, especially the green leafy ones, alfalfa, barley, and avocados.

When the body lacks vitamin B6, the following symptoms can occur: pins and needles in the legs, dizziness, nausea, anemia, nervous disorders such as confusion, spasms, and convulsions (like in epilepsy), edema, greenish urine, fat and cholesterol problems, skin infections, oral sores, alopecia, and seborrhea.

Vitamin B6 has no toxic side effects, as it is water-soluble, and is excreted in the urine, but very large doses can induce nervous disorders, bad dreams, and disturbed sleep, so the daily amount should not exceed 500 mg.

Vitamin B10

Vitamin B10 is commonly known as folic acid or folacin. It is also called vitamin B9, B11, and other names. The name "folic acid" derives from the Latin word for leaf, folium, because folic acid was initially produced from green leaves. Folic acid plays several important roles in metabolism, including the synthesis and breakdown of fibrinogen, which is involved in blood clotting. When foods that contain folic acid are cooked, up to half of the folic acid is destroyed.

Megaloblastic anemia is linked to a lack of folic acid, and there is also a link to a lack of white blood cells.

Vitamin B12 and folic acid can replace each other, if one of them is lacking - but we don't yet know how this works.

These two vitamins together produce the coenzyme required for breaking down and using protein.

Folic acid has many important functions: It plays an active part in the division of DNA. If there is a shortage of it in the body during pregnancy, the fetus could suffer from birth defects. In conjunction with vitamin C, folic acid has been known to inhibit certain kinds of cancer. It prevents macrocytic anemia, and helps exploit and synthetize amino acids. It helps in cell generation, and the production of red blood cells. It combats intestinal parasites and food poisoning, and enhances breast-feeding.

It is good for maintaining healthy skin and hair - in fact, in conjunction with PABA (para-aminobenzoic acid) and vitamin B5, it combats the graying of the hair. It both stimulates and inhibits the appetite. It alleviates heartburn, oral infections, and digestive problems.

The amount of folic acid required by the body is measured in micrograms (mcg). The recommended average daily amount for children up to six months is 30 mcg, for children up to one year, 45 mcg, for children up to tyree years, 100 mcg, and for youngsters up to 18 years, 400 mcg. For adults, it ranges between 400 and 500 mcg, according to the physical situation. Factors such as anemia, medication, pregnancy, etc., must be taken into account. For instance, pregnant women, and people who are taking large doses of vitamin C must take more folic acid. In general, multi-vitamin or B-complex tablets provide 400 mcg of folic acid per tablet.

What are the sources of folic acid? The following foods contain folic acid: liver, dried brewer's yeast, torula yeast, wheat-germ, soy flour, bran, dry chickpeas, nuts, beans, almonds, sunflower seeds, alfalfa, raw spinach, and all leafy vegetables. There is a small amount of folic acid in mother's milk and cow's milk.

If there is a shortage of folic acid in the body, the following symptoms can occur: Macrocytic anemia, in which the red blood cells are abnormally large, and contain less hemoglobin than normal; slow growth; digestive disorders, including diarrhea and nausea; a slippery red tongue and tongue infections; graying hair; mental problems, depression, sleeplessness, loss of appetite, fatigue; convulsions from birth, harelip; skin problems.

Folic acid has no toxic side-effects. However, some people experience skin allergies in the form of itching.

Vitamin B12

Vitamin B12 is also known as cyanocobalamin or hydroxycobalamin. It is the only compound in the living organism that contains cobalt - hence the name. Measured in micrograms (mcg), it is found in the form of cobalamin concentrate in tablets and food. Although the structure of vitamin B12 was identified in 1955, and the symptoms of B12 shortage were known many years before that, it was only in 1977 that it was produced synthetically.

Hydroxycobalamin is broken down by vitamin C when both are present in the stomach. This form is more widespread also when vitamin B12 is taken in the form of shots, since it remains in the body longer and with fewer health risks than shots of cyanocobalamin.

Vitamin B12 is synthetized in the intestines in the presence of a kind of protein called "extrinsic factor," which attaches itself to B12 and enables it to be absorbed in the intestines. B12 is found mainly in natural food, and for this reason is also known as "the red vitamin." B12 interacts well with the other B vitamins. Balanced action of the thyroid gland helps in the assimilation and absorption of B12.

Vitamin B12 performs the following functions in the body: It is essential for the formation of red blood cells, and, together with other B vitamins, prevents anemia. Together with B1 and B5, it is needed for the production of insulin and gall secretion. It enhances the action of folic acid and iron.

It is important for the efficient functioning of the nervous system, bone marrow, and all the cells. Vitamin B12 is needed for the production of nucleic acid and the exchange of amino acids.

It plays an important role in the metabolism of protein, fats, and carbohydrates. It helps people who suffer from allergies, asthma, and post-allergic conditions, as well as psychotic disorders, agitation, forgetfulness, and manic-depressive psychosis.

It improves memory, concentration, and cerebral balance. Moreover, it enhances growth in children, and stimulates the appetite. It combats body odor and backache. It is an important component in a number of enzymes of the nerve tissues (including the nerves of the spinal cord).

The recommended average daily amount for infants up to six months is 0.5 mcg, for children up to one year, 1.5 mgc, for children up to 3 years, 2 mcg, for youngsters up to 18 years, 3 mcg (optimal dose).

For adults, it is 3 mcg (more during pregnancy), although between 5 and 2,000 mcg can be taken, depending on the individual's physical condition. Vitamin B12 should be combined with folic acid and other B vitamins. People with a protein-rich diet need to take a greater amount of vitamin B12. Calcium should be taken in conjunction with B12 in order to make the absorption more efficient; vitamin C is also necessary.

Where can vitamin B12 be found? Eating the following foods will provide vitamin B12: beef, liver, inner organs, eggs, dairy products (cheeses), pickled or fermented vegetables, such as sauerkraut, and tofu (from soybeans).

A lack of vitamin B12 can cause the following symptoms: pernicious anemia; a swollen tongue, debility, weight loss, and tickling in the limbs; irregularities in walking, that sometimes begin with odd sensations and tickling in the fingers and toes; disappearance or aggravation of the nervous reflexes in the knees or Achilles tendon.

The reasons for a shortage of vitamin B12, besides not eating the right kinds of food, include excessive drinking at meals, alcohol, estrogen (in the Pill or in hormone treatment), acids and bases, and sleeping pills.

Vitamin B12 has no toxic side-effects, even in megadoses.

Vitamin B13

Vitamin B13 is also called orotic acid, and it is involved in the exchange of vitamin B12 and folic acid. Like all the other B vitamins, it is water-soluble, which means that it is destroyed by both water and light.

Very little is known about this vitamin, other than that it is important for children, and it is found in vegetables, especially root vegetables, as well as in whey. It is helpful in treating multiple sclerosis, as well as in avoiding certain liver problems, and some of the symptoms of aging.

The consequences of a shortage of vitamin B13 have not yet been determined, nor, unfortunately, have the recommended daily amounts. However, the vitamin has been called calcium orotate, and it should be taken only under the supervision of a physician or a naturopath.

Vitamin B15

Although no definitive research has been conducted on water-soluble vitamin B15, it is considered to part of the vitamin B group. Russian scientists, who have performed the bulk of vitamin B15 research, claim that it operates as an anti-oxidant in a manner similar to vitamin E, so it works best with vitamin A or E. Vitamin B15 is also known as pangamic acid and other names.

Vitamin B15 increases the efficient use of oxygen in the body, and improves and increases the life of the cells. It regulates the amount of steroids in the body (this is focus of the research by sports figures in Russia). It neutralizes the craving for alcohol, and accelerates the recovery from fatigue and exhaustion. It is effective in the treatment of stomach ulcers and shingles, and decreases the amount of cholesterol. It alleviates the symptoms of angina pectoris, asthma, and emphysema. It is important for the metabolism of protein, fats and sugars, and for this reason it plays a significant role in diabetes and arterial sclerosis. It protects the liver from cirrhosis by preventing fat from being filtered into it. It improves the reactions of the immune system, and is important in places where there is a low level of oxygen, or severe air pollution.

Insufficient research has been performed in order to know exactly what the results of a B15 deficiency are, but it seems that heart problems, nervous disorders, asthma, glaucoma, and liver problems (such as cirrhosis, infection and hepatitis) occur when B15 is lacking.

To date, there are no recommended daily amounts, except by physician's or naturopath's prescription. Vitamin B15 is mainly given to (Russian) sportsmen and athletes. B15 comes in 50 mg tablets, which should be taken after a heavy meal. Foods that contain B15 include whole grains (whole-wheat flour, brown rice, ground whole sesame seeds), brewer's yeast, and pumpkin seeds.

No toxicity has been reported, since B15 is not commercially distributed, but some young athletes have reported a feeling of nausea after taking large doses.

Vitamin B17

Vitamin B17 is also called amygdalin and other names, and it is a compound of two sugar molecules - benzaldehyde plus cyanide. B17 is a controversial vitamin, because practitioners of alternative medicine claim that it plays a role in cancer treatment. While the FDA in the United States does not recognize it, half of the states in the US permit its use, as do Mexico and many European countries. In fact, research done in those places shows success in the treatment of cancer with vitamin B17.

Vitamin B17 is produced from apricot pits, and is used as a prophylaxis against cancer. Nutritionists worldwide recommend eating between five and thirty apricot pits a day (not all at once) in order to increase one's life force. The principal aim of vitamin B17 is controlling cancer. It is used as a treatment for cancer, under the supervision of a physician or a naturopath.

There is no official recommended dose, but it comes in pills ranging between 0.25 and 1.0 grams, and one gram should be taken a day. Vitamin B17 can be found in the following foods: apricot, peach, plum, cherry, apple and pear pits - but the fruit must be organic, otherwise you will be consuming the pesticides that accumulate in the pits! Vitamin B17 is the only B vitamin that is not found in brewer's yeast.

Up until now, no specific symptoms resulting from a lack of vitamin B17 have been discovered. Having said that, it seems to have a general positive effect on life force and resistance to cancer.

There are no toxic side-effects in vitamin B17. However, it may only be taken under supervision, and the usual dose is one gram. A maximum of three grams may be taken, but at intervals during the day.

Inositol

Inositol, a water-soluble member of the vitamin B complex, is considered to be lipotropic, which means that it is essential for the metabolism of fat. It works with choline as a component of lecithin and as a cerebral neurotransmitter component. As with many of the other B vitamins, inositol is destroyed during the processing of food, by alcohol, caffeine, hormones, and medications such as sleeping pills. Of all the B vitamins, children's bodies contain the most lecithin and inositol.

The functions of inositol include helping to lower high cholesterol levels; maintaining healthy hair and skin, and protecting against eczema; providing the brain cells with nutrition; safeguarding bone marrow; protecting the liver against sclerosis; speeding up intestinal peristalsis; and safeguarding the intestinal cells.

There are no limitations in the recommended daily amount of inositol. However, it should be taken in conjunction with equal amounts of choline. The recommended average daily amount for children, especially chocolate eaters and/or cola drinkers (which contain caffeine) is 50-100 mg. For adults, it ranges between 250 and 500 mg.

Inositol can be found in the following foods: liver, lecithin (mainly from soybeans), brewer's yeast, whole wheat, wheatgerm, molasses, dry lima beans, peanuts, cabbage, yams, oranges, grapefruit, and melons.

The following symptoms may be manifested if there is a lack of inositol: eczema, hair loss, constipation, high cholesterol level, peculiar phenomena in the eye.

To date, inositol has not been found to have either side-effects or toxicity.

Biotin

Biotin is a water-soluble vitamin that is destroyed by oxidation. It is important for the metabolism of proteins and fats, and plays a role in the production of (essential) fatty acids, and helps utilize folic acid, and vitamins B5 and B12. Biotin is also called vitamin H (from the German word, Haut, meaning "skin"), or coenzyme R, and is measured in micrograms (mcg). A lack of biotin leads to a red, scaly skin condition called erythma. Biotin is neutralized by antibiotics, as well as by a substance called evadin, which is present in raw or insufficiently cooked egg yolks. The biotin disappears because the bacteria that synthetize it in the large intestine are destroyed. The result is alopecia (hair loss). Biotin is also necessary for the synthesis of ascorbic acid (vitamin C).

In a balanced diet, enough biotin is synthetized to enhance and be enhanced by vitamins A, B2, B3 and B6. If the intestinal flora have been damaged by antibiotics, biotin will be destroyed, and its action halted.

Biotin functions in the following ways: It is vital for the production of glycogen, nucleic acid, and amino acids. It participates in the production of white blood cells (T-cells) and antibodies. It maximizes the use of vitamin B12, vitamin B5 and folic acid. It protects the hair from graying and falling out, and is effective against baldness. It regulates the level of saturated fats (and therefore also of cholesterol). It alleviates muscle pains, muscle cramps, and "growing pains." It treats conditions of eczema and dermatitis.

The recommended average daily dose for children up to

four years is 150 mcg, and for youngsters up to 18 years is 300 mcg. For adults, it ranges between 25 and 300 mcg per day. Therapeutic doses can be as high as 800 mcg per day - sometimes even more.

It is interesting that the amount of biotin in mother's milk increases a week post-partum.

In which foodstuffs can biotin be found? In dried brewer's yeast, ox liver, nuts, egg yolks, milk, brown rice, and most fruit.

If there is a shortage of biotin in the body, the following symptoms may occur: metabolic disturbances and disruption of the folic acid supply; eczema, skin infections, and gray skin; hair loss; swollen tongue; muscle pains; loss of appetite, nausea; apathy.

No toxicity has been found in biotin - either in children or in adults.

Choline

Choline belongs to the lipotropic group which also includes methionine, betaine, and inositol, with which choline is closely linked. Choline is found in all the cells of the body, and, as it is part of acetylcholine, plays a vital role in the neurotransmitters (the chemical substance that transmits messages from one nerve to another). It is therefore very important for the brain and memory. Choline helps prevent the formation of gallstones, since it is connected to dissolving cholesterol, and prevents the blockage of arteries. Choline, which is part of lecithin, prevents the accumulation of fats in the liver, and helps to rid the liver of toxins. Moreover, it is important for myelin, which is the substance that forms the medullary sheath of nerve-fibers.

Choline is one of the few substances that has access to the brain cells, and it also serves as a raw material for the hormones of the thyroid gland, and so, in addition to its functions as a fat solvent, it helps prevent excessive weight-gain. Choline is destroyed by sulfa, estrogen (in the form of the Pill or hormones), alcohol, industrial food-processing, and excessive drinking.

In addition to the functions mentioned above, choline also helps with the metabolism of fats; helps in the synthesis of hormones such as epinephrine; dissolves surplus cholesterol and triglycerides; serves as a medication for cirrhosis of the liver, and is important in the treatment of other diseases such as ulcers, Alzheimer's, high blood pressure, low sugar, psoriasis, and heart and kidney ailments.

There are no clear-cut recommended daily amounts, but children should definitely receive 500 to 900 mg of choline per day, while adults require 1,000 mg. When used as a specific treatment, the dosage is greater, whether the supplement is choline or lecithin (which breaks down into choline and inositol in the body). It should be remembered that when taking large doses of lecithin, calcium and magnesium should also be taken.

The foods in which choline can be found are: liver, kidneys, brains, egg yolks, green vegetables, brewer's yeast, wheat-germ, lecithin, dried peas, dried beans, soybeans, whole-wheat flour, and oats.

If there is a lack of choline in the body, the following symptoms may occur: renal bleeding, problems with the heart muscle, cirrhosis and excess fat in the liver, arterial sclerosis, and a possible link to Alzheimer's.

Choline has no known toxicity; however, if it is taken for an extended period, vitamin B6 should also be taken, and as with the whole B vitamin group, B complex (including B6).

Water-soluble PABA

Water-soluble PABA belongs to the vitamin B complex, and is also called vitamin BX. It is produced in the intestines by the intestinal bacteria; in conjunction with these bacteria, it helps produce folic acid - and this accounts for its importance in the production of red blood cells.

PABA has been proven to be linked to the reduction of the risk of skin cancer, maintains skin color, and creates resistance against sunburn. For this reason, PABA is used for treating vitiligo (white patches on the skin), eczema, and white patches on the skin. It also helps prevent bad breath and body odor, mainly in conjunction with vitamin B6, zinc, and magnesium.

PABA is produced by the intestinal flora, and is destroyed by antibiotics, which destroy the flora, by industrial food processing, by sulfa and estrogen, and by alcohol.

In addition to the functions of PABA mentioned above, PABA also reduces the pain resulting from burns, protects skin and hair color, enhances the influences of pantothenic acid (vitamin B5), and assists in the production of folic acid.

There are no clear-cut average daily amounts, and if the digestive system and intestinal flora are in good condition, there is no real need for PABA supplements, especially since it is found in every vitamin B complex formula. Adults require between 30 and 100 mg per day. However, this dosage should be increased if the person is taking penicillin, sulfa drugs, or the Pill. PABA can be found in the following foodstuffs: dry brewer's yeast, whole untoasted grains, brown rice, bran, wheat-germ, molasses, liver, and kidneys.

If there is a lack of PABA in the body, the following symptoms can occur - fatigue, nervousness, and headaches; constipation, digestive problems; eczema, skin problems, and hair loss; anemia and loss of libido; scleroderma (hardening of the skin).

PABA has not been found to have any toxic effects; having said that, large doses should not be taken for any length of time without medical supervision. Pre-toxic symptoms include nausea and vomiting.

Vitamin C

This vitamin is known by several names, including ascorbic acid, calcium ascorbate, and cevitamin acid. With the exception of human beings, monkeys and guinea-pigs, most animals produce vitamin C in their bodies, in a proportion of 45 mg per kilogram of body weight.

Even though as early as 1747, Dr. Lind gave citrus fruit to seamen as a very effective method of combating scurvy, the vitamin was isolated as a compound only in 1928, and was synthetized for the first time in 1934. Scurvy was in fact described by the ancient Greek physician, Hippocrates. It occurred mainly in seafarers, who spent long months at sea, and, lacking refrigeration facilities, were deprived of fresh fruit and vegetables (especially citrus fruit) in their diet.

Like many other vitamins, there is a controversy as to the daily amount that should be taken. Researchers in the vitamin and mineral field have overwhelmingly ruled that ten times the dose recommended by the RDA should be taken. As it is water-soluble, it is not stored in the body in its natural form. Surplus vitamin C is excreted in the urine.

Vitamin C plays an important role in tissue-building in the body: cartilaginous collagen, teeth, and bones. It is also linked to the production of interferon, and is among the "leaders" of the immune system, exterminating bacteria, and thus fighting viral and bacterial infections. It catalyzes the healing of wounds and helps stop internal bleeding.

Vitamin C helps the body to filter out various poisons, and so people who are subjected to air pollution, including cigarette smoke, or suffer from tension of various kinds, must increase their daily intake of vitamin C.

Since its discovery, extensive literature has been written about it, and vast research conducted, showing vitamin C's effectiveness in therapeutic doses in respiratory tract problems such as asthma, sinusitis, bronchitis, aural infections, and so on, and other serious diseases such as cardiac infarction, thromboses, blood vessel disorders, fertility problems in men - right up to all kinds of cancer in both men and women.

In addition to the very important functions described above, vitamin C prevents premature degeneration of the body by preventing oxidation of the cells. It plays a role in the formation of hormones (in their synthesis), as well as in the production of red blood cells and the absorption of iron from the intestines. Since vitamin C forms part of the nutrition of the nervous system, it is important in states of stress.

The fact that it produces collagen means that it helps in the healing of tissues, and in the congealing of wounds. However, it also reduces blood crystallization that can cause blockages in veins. In conjunction with other minerals such as zinc and selenium, vitamin C eliminates toxicity from metals and chemical pollution, and as such is important after surgery.

Most people know that vitamin C is effective when they have colds or flu, and in fact, more than that, the vitamin is effective with general respiratory problems, as well as allergies and sensitivities. Vitamin C is used to prevent SIDS (cradle death).

As was mentioned above, it plays a crucial role in the prevention of scurvy, as well as gum problems. It enhances the treatment of mononucleosis, colitis (inflammation of the intestine), and generally of all infections. In high doses, it is effective in relieving constipation. Vitamin C reduces cholesterol.

The RDA recommends 35-45 mg of vitamin C per day for children up to 10 years, 50 mg for youngsters up to 14, and 60 mg for people from 15 years onward. This amount is ludicrous, and should be ignored, since it was determined half a century ago. Today, the recommended average daily amount of vitamin C for children up to one year is about 35 mg, for children up to ten years is 100 mg, and for youngsters up to 18 years is 500 mg. Adults require at least 500 mg per day. Larger doses than those mentioned above are given therapeutically, or to women on the Pill or undergoing hormone treatment.

The intake of vitamin C should be divided up during the day, as it is expelled with the urine every 2-3 hours. A solution to this problem is to take Time-Release C tablets, which releases the vitamin gradually. These tablets are also known as C-ester.

Where can vitamin C be found? It can be found in the following foods: citrus fruits such as grapefruit, lemons, oranges (and their juice), and tangerines, other fruits such as black currants, guavas, mangoes, papayas and strawberries, in vegetables such as broccoli, brussels sprouts, cabbage, spinach, watercress, collard and kale, in green, sweet, and hot peppers, in potatoes, and in tomatoes and rose hips.

If there is a lack of vitamin C, the following symptoms may occur: scurvy, which manifests itself in rapid fatigue during effort, bleeding gums, bleeding muscles and joints, pains in the joints - to the point of death.

As for toxicity, natural vitamin C is not toxic, as any surplus of the vitamin is excreted during urination.

However, synthetic vitamin C (ascorbic acid) should not be taken in doses exceeding three tablets a day. Larger doses can cause diarrhea, excessive urination, and itchy skin. In megadoses, there is a danger of kidney-stone formation if magnesium is not taken concurrently.

It is preferable to use natural vitamin C, especially in the form that includes the whole vitamin C complex (with bioflavonoids), as is explained in the next section.

Vitamin P

Vitamin P includes the following components: the bioflavonoids, rutin, hesperidin and quarcetin, which constitute the family of the vitamin C complex, along with over 30 other substances, such as citrin, flavones, and flonals. Most of the properties of the bioflavonoids are similar to those of vitamin C, and in fact, the two groups support each other. In nature, they always occur together. Fortunately, the vitamin P group has not yet been manufactured synthetically, unlike ascorbic acid, so if you take a vitamin C supplement, you should take C complex which is a compound of natural vitamins P and C.

Bioflavonoids operate in the capillaries, and one of their functions is to prevent the accumulation and congestion of blood cells, just as vitamin C does in the veins and arteries, and just as rutin operates in the larger blood vessels. The action of the entire vitamin P group is thinning the blood so that it can flow through all the body's capillaries and cells (without needing aspirin, which, in all its forms, stimulates the flow of blood). Like vitamin C, bioflavonoids are destroyed by water, industrial food processing, heat, light and smoke.

What are the functions of bioflavonoids? Well, in overall terms, since they are part of the vitamin C family, their action is the same as that of vitamin C. They prevent bleeding gums, they provide immunity against infections, and they enhance the operation of vitamin C, and increase its effectiveness; they strengthen the capillaries and blood vessels. Very importantly, they prevent the conversion of surplus glucose into sorbitol (a crystalline substance that resembles corn sugar), thus preventing damage to the capillaries in diabetics. Moreover, they are helpful in the treatment of dizziness that derives from problems in the balancing mechanism in the inner ear.

The recommended average daily amount for children is 100 mg (as part of vitamin C complex), and for adults is 500 mg (as part of vitamin C complex).

Bioflavonoids can be found in the following foods: fruit and vegetables, in the white layer that lies below the peel of citrus fruit, and in the fleshy part of peppers where the seeds are found, in plums, cherries, strawberries, apricots, rose hips, grapes, and buckwheat.

We must remember that if fruit and vegetables are sprayed with pesticides (and grapes are sprayed to an extent that is mind-boggling), most of the vitamin C and bioflavonoids are used up neutralizing the pesticides themselves rather than benefiting our bodies. This means that anyone who wants to obtain his daily supply of vitamins from fruit and vegetables should only eat those that are organically grown (without pesticides and other chemical treatments).

If there is a lack of bioflavonoids, the symptoms that can occur are similar to those of a lack of vitamin C, in addition to capillary fragility.

Just like vitamin C, bioflavonoids are not toxic.

Vitamin D

Vitamin D is also known as calciferol, ergosterol, and the "sun vitamin", and sometimes also ergocalciferol or cholecalciferol.

In 1923, it transpired that it was possible to cure rickets (a disease in which the bones soften and become deformed) by ultraviolet irradiation of ergosterol to the skin, thus transforming a substance in the outer layer of skin (dihydrotachysterol) into vitamin D. In 1924, it was discovered that this compound, which could prevent rickets, had a special chemical structure - called a sterol structure - which is the basic structure of all hormones and cholesterol. The term "vitamin D" is an inclusive name for the family which includes: vitamins D1, D2, D3, D4 and D5.

Vitamin D1 only has a historic value, which is the results of ergosterol irradiation. Vitamin D2 is the synthetic product that is similar, with slight differences, to vitamin D3. Vitamin D3 is the natural product, which is actually vitamin D. Vitamins D4 and D5 are produced by sterol irradiation, and have no therapeutic value.

Vitamin D is oil-soluble (as are vitamins A, E and K), and it is stored mainly in the liver, as well as in the brain, the spleen, and the bones, after being formed by exposure to sunlight or by nutrition. This vitamin is vital for bones and teeth, as well as for calcium and phosphorus absorption.

As it is oil-soluble, our body requires natural oil in which there are unsaturated fatty acids (cold-pressed). Mineral oil destroys vitamin D.

In addition to rickets, in which the bones soften and

become deformed, this vitamin is important for all bone and calcium problems, such as osteoporosis, and damage to the teeth. Since the air we breathe is not pure - it contains soot, smoke, and so on - sunlight does not reach our skin properly when we sunbathe, so the natural production of vitamin D is disrupted. The use of synthetic soaps that remove all the fatty layers from the skin (in our eternal quest to be clean!) also causes a situation in which sunlight cannot come into contact with the good fat on our skins in order to convert it into vitamin D, so there is almost nothing useful about sunbathing. Of course, we should never overexpose our bodies to the sun, or get sunburned, because of the risk of skin cancer. To top it all off, the use of sunscreens halts the production of vitamin D.

The functions of vitamin D include strengthening the bones and teeth (along with calcium and magnesium). It is also helpful with conjunctivitis, and, along with vitamins A and C, helps prevent colds. It assists in the absorption and assimilation of vitamin A, and is good for enzyme production. It is useful in the treatment of skin ailments such as acne and psoriasis, and alleviates allergies and pains in the joints.

The recommended average daily amounts (found in supplements) of vitamin D are 100-400 IU for adults, and 100 IU for children. These amounts have been found to be beneficial.

Where is vitamin D found? In fish, such as salmon, tuna and herring, in dairy products, in egg yolks, in fish oil (which also comes in the form of tablets), and in carp oil.

In the event of a lack of vitamin D, the following symptoms may occur: rickets in children, osteoporosis and osteomalacia (softening of the bones), problems with teeth, including decay and breakdown, retarded growth in children, elongated skull, constipation, problems with vision, and muscle weakness.

Taken in normal doses, there is no problem of toxicity with vitamin D. However, in large doses,, it can be toxic to certain people. Megadoses are considered to be toxic, resulting in vomiting, severe thirst, burning eyes, itchy skin, and diarrhea. In the normal course of things, however, there is nothing to worry about, since such an amount is equivalent to over 100 vitamin D tablets - which is an entire bottle meant to be one to three months' supply!

Vitamin E

Although vitamin E can be called the "omnipotent vitamin," and it is considered one of the most important for human beings (and there is no such thing as an unimportant vitamin), the funny thing is that this vitamin was discovered as a result of research involving rats, after reproductive disturbances were traced to the lack of particular factors in the foods that they had been fed.

Vitamin E was discovered in 1922, when, in the research that was being performed, it was thought at first that reproductive disturbances, both in male and female rats (to the point of sterility), stemmed from poisoning, and only afterward did it transpire that the disturbances were the result of a lack. When it was discovered, the factor was called "tocopherol" (tokos means "birth" in Greek), and only in 1936 was the vitamin successfully isolated from wheat-germ oil. Today, eight types of tocopherols are produced from plant oils.

It is very important to take vitamin E when taking iron supplements, so as to improve the absorption of the iron. Vitamin E is plays an important role in the absorption and assimilation of iron, even though its action is not yet clear.

Vitamin E is oil-soluble and is measured in IU, with each unit being the equivalent of one mg. As was mentioned above, there are eight types of tocopherols: alpha, beta, gamma, delta, epsilon, zeta, eta, and theta (according to the first eight letters of the Greek alphabet).

The most effective of all is alpha-tocopherol. (The substance that is called d-alpha-tocopherol is the natural one, while d-l-alpha-tocopherol is the synthetic one, and is not recommended.)

Because it is an anti-oxidant (like vitamins A and C, and selenium), it lowers the fat and cholesterol levels in the blood, and because of its additional properties as a substance that decreases the viscosity of the drops of blood, it is used for reducing heart diseases and for strengthening the heart muscle. Research (among the biggest ever performed in the world) was conducted on vitamin E in which it was proved that the longer vitamin E is taken, the fewer heart attacks will occur, and the lower the risk.

The recommended RDA dosage ranges from 3-4 mg (IU) in infants up to 1 year, to 10-30 mg (IU) in adults, but in almost every (therapeutic) case, it is recommended that the initial dosage be at least double that. People with high blood pressure or damaged heart valves should take less than a person with normal blood pressure. People who suffer from low blood pressure can and should take natural vitamin E in higher quantities (under medical supervision), since it balances the blood pressure. Research has also shown that vitamin E is effective in the cure and prevention of cancer.

Vitamin E also exists in both powder form and in a water-soluble form. Their strength is about half of that of natural vitamin E (oil-soluble).

Water-soluble vitamin E is recommended for people suffering from an inability to break down fats because of a liver or a gall-bladder problem.

Additional functions of vitamin E are to reduce acidity and the oxidation of cells, and to protect all the oil-soluble vitamins (A, D and K). In conjunction with vitamin C, it is useful in preventing thromboses (blood clots). Moreover, it helps in providing oxygen to the cells (for breathing), especially of the muscles. It reduces the turnover of red blood cells, and helps prevent and eliminate scars and many other skin problems. It protects and helps in the formation of the hormones of the adrenal glands, the pituitary gland, and the sex hormones.

It is helpful in female fertility (including problems for which hormones are prescribed as solutions), and also in male fertility, in which a lack of vitamin E leads to problems with sperm cells. It is effective in safeguarding pregnancies and in preventing birth defects.

It also helps cure tics of various kinds, as well as internal and external infections. As we mentioned earlier, it is important for the absorption of iron. It protects against toxins and emetics.

In which foods can vitamin E be found? In whole grains (whole wheat, brown rice), wheat-germ (and wheat-germ oil), corn and soy oil (cold-pressed only), in most vegetable oils (cold-pressed only), eggs, broccoli, bean sprouts, spinach, soy, and green leafy vegetables.

If there is a lack of vitamin E, the following symptoms may occur: There may be muscle weakness, leading to the person being cross-eyed as a result of weakness in the muscles of the eye. It can cause muscle degeneration, as well as swelling and destruction of muscles. A lack of vitamin E can cause impaired metabolism of fats. Related to this are problems with cholesterol and triglycerides. There could be damage to blood vessels (veins), and angina pectoris. Blood conditions such as phlebitis and thromboses could occur. There could be phenomena of sterility and a lack of sperm motility. Diseases such as cancer, diabetes, arthritis, and retarded growth in children may also occur.

In principle, vitamin E is not toxic, and the warnings about the amounts stem from the fact of its being a regulator of blood pressure. People who suffer from a lack of vitamin K are forbidden to take large quantities of vitamin E, since this is liable to cause blockages in the blood vessels. (A shortage of vitamin K is connected to blood clotting.)

Vitamin F

The truth of the matter is that vitamin F is not a vitamin at all; it is just a collective name for unsaturated fatty acids, which are the essential fats: linoleic and linolenic acids. Vitamin F is measured in milligrams. There are no RDA guidelines for these fatty acids, but there is a recommendation that one percent of the daily calorie intake consist of these acids.

What does vitamin F do? It helps burn up saturated fats, and is divided into two main groups: Omega 3, which is found more in fish fats (from the north), and is also called EPA/DHA, and Omega 6, which is found in plants. The fatty acids mentioned above are distilled and extracted from regular fats in the processing procedure, which renders regular fats (which are not cold-pressed) worthless from this point of view. Vitamin F is used in the treatment of every case of skin problems, acne and eczema (including psoriasis), and is used in practically every treatment for lowering the cholesterol in the blood.

These fatty acids (vitamin F) are destroyed by excess saturated fats, by heat and by oxidation. (See the explanation of fats on page 62.)

What is the role of vitamin F in our bodies? Well, it helps in the prevention of anemia; it also keeps the hair and skin healthy, and, in conjunction with PABA and pantothenic acid, slows down the graying of the hair. It is helpful in the growth of children by enabling calcium to be absorbed in the cells. It maintains the weight at a steady level by burning saturated fats. It improves the quality of mother's milk. It protects against intestinal parasites (including Candida albicans). It is especially helpful during PMS, as well as in menstrual problems.

There are no recommended daily amounts, but it is a good idea to include polyunsaturated fatty acids, to the amount of one percent, in the daily calorie intake. Children (and adults, too, for that matter) who consume large amounts of carbohydrates, should take a large amount.

When there is a problem of a lack of vitamin F, the amounts should be increased - under the supervision of a physician, a naturopath, or a dietician who understands the principles of food supplements.

Where can vitamin F be found? In the form of Omega 3, in oil from northern fish, EPA/DHA, which also comes in capsules. In the form of Omega 6 - in vegetable oils (only cold-pressed): wheat-germ oil, pumpkin seed oil, sunflower oil, corn oil, safflower oil, soy oil, almond oil and other nut oils - except for brazil and cashew nuts.

Especially rich oils are evening primrose oil, which is available both in capsule and in the form of drops, blackberry oil, which is found in capsules, and fox-tail oil, which comes in capsule form.

If there is a shortage of vitamin F, the following symptoms could occur: acne, eczema and other skin problems, such as psoriasis. Women could suffer from PMS in the form of cramps and irritability.

No toxicity has been found in any form of vitamin F.

Fats

All the fats derived from animal sources are saturated fats, except for fish oil.

Olive oil, almond oil, and avocado oil all contain mono-unsaturated fatty acids, and the rest of the oils, as was mentioned previously, are polyunsaturated, and these are the oils we need more.

Cold-pressed oils should not be used for frying; they should be added to food - to salads, rice, etc. - since during frying, the spatial structure of the oil changes (cis/trans) and, just like saturated oil, it becomes a negative health factor that presents a risk of arterial sclerosis, high blood pressure, cholesterol, and so on.

When a person consumes fats (good ones polyunsaturated), linolenic acid partially turns into the gamma form, from which the body's hormones (prostaglandins) are built. If these hormones are lacking, the problems mentioned above occur. Evening primrose oil (like blackberry oil and fox-tail oil) contains the gamma form of linolenic acid, and the body activates it immediately, both for creating prostaglandins and for myelin, the substance that forms the medullary sheath of nerves.

Vitamin K

The name of this vitamin comes from the word coagulation, because of its important role in the blood coagulation process. Between 1920 and 1930, the various substances that were called K1, K2 and K3 were investigated in order to examine cases in which there were problems in blood coagulation.

Vitamin K is also called menadione, and occasionally phytonadione as a supplement in baby food, and is measured in micrograms (mcg). The K1 and K2 forms are natural, while K3 is synthetic.

Vitamin D is necessary in the liver in order to convert the protein prothrombin into thrombin, which is the blood coagulation factor. If there is insufficient vitamin K, thrombin will not be formed, and blood coagulation will be impaired.

Vitamin K is synthetized in the intestines and supplied to the body by the consumption of green vegetables. There is almost no need for a supply of vitamin K from external sources or pills, except in cases in which there is a problem of absorption in the intestines, or if the intestinal flora has been damaged.

Vitamin K is destroyed by X-rays, air pollution, freezing (of food), aspirins, and medications. In recent years, we have found increasing damage to the intestinal flora as a result of the excessive use of antibiotics and a lack of awareness that acidophilus must be administered with or after antibiotics (if there really is a need for them).

The intestinal fungus Candida albicans has also become a serious problem (even if for some reason many doctors ignore it), and this is because of antibiotics and hormones - those in the Pill as well as those "supplied" to the public, whether it wants them or not, in chicken, meat, eggs, and milk.

The functions of vitamin K include, in addition to its role in blood coagulation, helping to prevent internal bleeding, hemorrhoids, and excessive bleeding during menstrual periods. Research has also shown that it has a serious effect in the fight against malignant tumors.

No more than 100 mcg vitamin K should be taken per day. If you take synthetic vitamin K, you can take up to 500 mcg per day. Recent research has shown that there is a connection between large supplementary doses of the vitamin and the acceleration of the onset of anemia.

Vitamin K is found in the following foods: yogurts, preferably those manufactured from sheep's or goat's milk, green vegetables, especially alfalfa sprouts, and also in the form of pills, egg yolks, cold-pressed safflower oil, fish oil, kelp, and molasses.

A vitamin K deficiency could cause the following: There could be internal or other kinds of hemorrhaging, including subcutaneous hemorrhages; blood coagulation could be impaired when an injury occurs. There is a risk of celiac disease (in which there is a sensitivity to gluten, the wheat protein), as well as colitis, and oral infections (sprue - a kind of infantile thrush).

No toxicity has been found in vitamin K, especially in its natural form.

Vitamin T

Vitamin T belongs to the group of vitamins that have not yet been sufficiently researched. This vitamin, like vitamin K, is also linked to blood coagulation, and it is connected with the blood platelets. For this reason, it is linked to anemia and to the various types of hemophilia. There is no vitamin T supplement in the form of pills; it is found only in food.

As was mentioned above, the main function of vitamin T is in blood coagulation and the movement of the platelets. In addition, it helps improve a weak memory.

Where is vitamin T found? In sesame seeds (for this reason, it is also sometimes called the "sesame vitamin"), and in egg yolks.

What happens if there is a lack of vitamin T in the body? Well, unfortunately, nobody really knows exactly, but there is a connection to hemophilia, which is a malfunction in the blood coagulation mechanism (it is a genetic/hereditary disease which is caused by the absence of two blood coagulation factors).

As yet, there are no recommended daily amounts, nor are there indications of toxicity.

Vitamin U

Very little is known about this vitamin, except that there is evidence of its role in controlling and healing ulcers.

There is no vitamin U supplement in the form of pills, and therefore there are no recommended daily amounts, or indications of toxicity.

Vitamin U is found in the vegetables of the cabbage family, such as cabbage, brussels sprouts, in cauliflower and kohlrabi. Its value in healing ulcers has been noted with the consumption of cabbage juices, and practical experience, including that of the author of this book, shows that drinking these juices, as part of an overall process, helps in healing of stomach and duodenal ulcers.

Coenzyme Q10

Coenzyme Q10, which is also known by other names, and is not a vitamin according to conventional definitions. Instead, it is considered to be essential to all the body's cells, tissues, and organs. Structurally, it resembles vitamin K, and is found in the cells of other animals and in plants. The heart and the liver contain the largest amount of co-enzyme Q10 in the body. Cardiac patients show a lack of up to 75% of the coenzyme.

Coenzyme Q10 is found in beef, sardines, spinach, and peanuts.

Coenzyme Q10 is essential for inhibiting or preventing destruction and "mechanical" action in the heart. It prevents problems in the coronary arteries, as well as infections and diseases of the muscles of the wall of the heart. Coenzyme Q10 is also useful in the treatment and prevention of angina pectoris, and in various forms of cardiac congestion: mitral valve cardio-myopathy, and hyperthyroid heart failure.

The coenzyme is helpful in regulating high blood pressure; it improves the energy, and has been shown to be important in the condition of chronic fatigue (the "Yuppie disease"). It improves the functioning of the immune system, which deteriorates over the years, and helps prevent viral or bacterial infections. The coenzyme is effective in treating gum problems - up to between 60 and 90 percent. It improves and strengthens resistance to various kinds of toxicity, including those caused by medications.

In diabetes, coenzyme Q10 helps lower the sugar level

by 20 to 30 percent. It helps when metabolism is weak. (Fifty percent of people who are obese apparently lack coenzyme Q10 in their bodies.)

Coenzyme Q10 has been found to be extremely important in the treatment of cancer and tumors.The recommended daily dosage of coenzyme Q10 (in therapeutic cases too) is 150-180 mg. In most cases, the dosage is decreased gradually. There are Q10 capsules of 10, 30, 50 and 60 mg respectively.

On an ongoing basis, the regular recommended dosage is 60 mg per day, which can be taken in the form of: 2X30 mg capsules, or 1X50 or 60 mg capsule per day.

As for toxicity, none has been found in co-enzyme Q10, but generally speaking, the daily dosage does not exceed 150 mg. Since the appropriate experiments have not yet been conducted, the coenzyme is not given to pregnant or nursing women.

This book attempts to emphasize the vital role played by vitamins in our health. So many diseases and conditions can be treated, cured or even avoided if we are aware of the contribution that vitamins make to our body's well-being, and ensure that our intake of them is regular and balanced.

No less important is the role of minerals. This fascinating and significant topic is dealt with in depth in another book in this series, called - appropriately - "Minerals."

Jon Tillman

Minerals

Introduction

The word "mineral" comes from "mine" - so it means a substance that is extracted from the earth.

The minerals that interest us are elements, which are primary, simple substances that constitute inorganic and organic bodies in nature, as well as in the human body. Minerals are the main components of certain parts of our bodies, such as teeth and bones (calcium), and they play an important role in the electrolytes (the electric transmitters), which are important for the normal functioning of the muscle and nervous systems, as well as for the body's balance or homeostasis.

All the minerals needed by and found in the body are contained in food, and are supplied, under normal circumstances, in the required form and quantity. Food must be the main supplier of the person's minerals, but under certain circumstances, it is necessary to take mineral supplements, mainly because of the absence of their organic form in modern foodstuffs. In addition, supplements are taken when it is necessary to use a mineral as an aid to the body - whether as a solution to a problem that requires a large quantity of the particular mineral, or in order to compensate for a substantial loss of the mineral from the body.

In this book, I will relate to each mineral in alphabetical order: its role in the body, children's and adults' daily requirements, in which natural sources (foodstuffs) it can be found, food supplements, and toxicity.

It is important to know the links between minerals and vitamins, and these will be indicated during the course of the book, but it must be remembered that the absorption of minerals by the digestive system is linked both to the acid-base balance, and to the combinations of minerals and proteins that require the presence of a protein in the mineral absorption process, and the presence of the appropriate digestive acid.

Minerals that are taken as food supplements must be bound to an amino acid (or some other organic link) in order to enable the mineral to be absorbed effectively.

Minerals that are bound to amino acids are called chealated minerals, and they are absorbed ten times better than minerals that are not bound to amino acids. Another important point is that only 10% of the quantity of non-organic minerals (used in the drug industry) are absorbed, as opposed to natural minerals.

Minerals

Aluminum

Chemical symbol Al, specific gravity 2.7, atomic weight 26.97 (alumen).

The most widespread metal in the earth's crust, its color resembles silver, it is light and convenient to shape, and for that reason it is used extensively in the disposable utensil industry and kitchen utensil industry (see further on).

For human beings, aluminum is a trace mineral that is also found in foodstuffs and natural food supplements. However, it is liable to cause harm and toxicity in the body.

Large quantities of aluminum have been found in the brains of people who died of Alzheimer's and Parkinson's diseases, and researchers believe that this is directly linked to the diseases (as are other toxicities), as a result of the absorption of the mineral into the tissues.

It is as yet unknown what the role - if any - of aluminum is in the human body, or if it is at all necessary. Nothing is known about a shortage of aluminum - only about excessive amounts. For this reason, there is no need to take any aluminum.

Toxicity is aluminum's major problem, and is manifested in the following (in addition to other as yet unknown problems):

Aluminum causes constipation and flatulence (your suspicions should be aroused when herbal remedies, dietary changes and/or medications and "natural medications" supplements don't help you). It also causes a tremor in the leg muscle, as well as excessive perspiration, and a loss of strength. The motor nerves can be paralyzed, and there can be a feeling of pins and needles. The absorption of phosphorus (which is necessary for calcium) is reduced, and this leads to bone and brain problems.

Aluminum is found in antacids; which also cause a shortage of vitamins A and B1, and other medications (alumina/magnesia), which also cause a shortage of iron and phosphates. When you take these medications (and you should always avoid doing so), you should also take brewer's yeast, cod-liver oil, (live) yogurt, and acidophilus with digestive enzymes.

Aluminum is also found in aluminum salts of fluorine, which are the enemies of fluorine itself. It is found in processed cheese, in aluminum pots and pans, and in aluminum products such as foil. The use of these objects causes aluminum to penetrate into the body. In summary, the use of cooking utensils and other aluminum products should be avoided entirely, especially in heating or cooking. Use stainless steel, glass, etc. instead. Consider this a warning!

Boron

Boron is one of the most recent minerals to date whose importance has been acknowledged.

Boron is found in food (vegetable), as are most of the minerals, and our bodies need small quantities of it. Boron's main property is that it is calcium's glue in the bones. However, in a great deal of research conducted in hospitals and research centers (mainly in the U.S.), the importance of boron in other fields is also being demonstrated.

Research conducted in 1987 indicates the importance of boron during the post-menopausal years, especially in the absorption of other minerals (in men, too). For this reason, it helps in the treatment of osteoporosis, since it enhances and catalyzes metabolic processes.

The need for boron was recognized in 1870, when the subject of borax/boric acid was investigated. For several decades afterwards, this substance was used as a preservative mainly for fish and meat, and, from the beginning of the 20th century, also for vegetables. It was found that in large quantities (as in preservatives), it is harmful, and therefore the use of borates in food for preservative purposes, which was common-place from the 1920s until the mid-1950s, was prohibited, mainly because of the various additives that converted it into boric acid, until the 1980s. In 1987, its importance was acknowledged once more, but not as a preservative.

Boron helps with the absorption of calcium, copper, and nitrogen. It increases the libido in post-menopausal women (because of the improvement in the concentration of testosterone in the blood). It helps in the treatment of cancer by enhancing the absorption of the other minerals. Boron helps in the absorption of zinc as well as of vitamin C (ascorbic acid), and has been found to be effective in treating and improving lung function.

Boron negates and prevents negative reactions in estrogen absorption, and in this way helps to reduce calcium loss and the increase in cholesterol and triglycerides as a result of the use of estrogen. It improves the metabolism for the absorption of calcium, and as such constitutes a factor for prevention and/or treatment of osteoporosis and arthritis. Boron raises the testosterone level in the blood threefold, thus enhancing muscle mass. It is necessary for growth (as are other trace minerals such as nickel, silicon, arsenic, cadmium, lithium, vanadium, and so on), apparently not as a direct factor, but rather as a link for calcium and other minerals.

Boron is helpful in curbing memory loss (a side-effect of aging) by stopping electro-encephalographic changes in the brain. It causes an increase in the copper concentration in the brain, as well as in the calcium concentration in the brain and the cortex - thus improving the memory. Boron is active and effective during menopause, especially for hot flashes and night sweats.

There is no daily recommended dietary allowance of boron, but research shows that the body requires no less than 1 mg per day, and up to 30 mg per day as an external supplement. The amount required by our bodies is up to 50 mg, some of which comes from food (if our diet is balanced).

A therapeutic amount of boron is about 3-6 mg, which

can be supplied in the form of 25-50 mg of borax decahydrate/sodium tetraborte. This amount is found in a combination supplement/tablet of calcium + magnesium + boron (the boron is 3 mg), and there is also a supplement/tablet of boron (3 mg) alone.

Boron can be found in the following foods: mainly plants, nuts, fruit and legumes, wine, dried fruit (raisins and prunes), broccoli, parsley, almonds, peanuts, apple juice and apple concentrate, cherries, the juice of organic grapes, canned peaches and pears. Boron is found less in animal products such as meat, poultry, fish, and dairy products.

It is easy to supply the body's boron needs (without using external means, except in a therapeutic situation) if the person knows how to plan and consume good (organic) foods.

Toxicity was discovered in research that was conducted on rats, dogs, pigs, and other animals. An amount of about 8 mg per kilogram body weight was found to be toxic (for example, if a person weighs 70 kg and takes 560 mg per day). Bigger amounts were found to cause damage in animals. The maximum amount (according to research) is 500 mg a day, an enormous amount that is almost impossible to consume.

Cadmium

Chemical symbol Cd, specific gravity 8.64, atomic weight 112.4 (cadmium).

Cadmium is a soft, gray-white metal. In nature, it is linked to minerals with zinc. In industry, it is used with other metals; moreover, it regulates the operation of atomic reactors. Cadmium salts are used for manufacturing yellow paints.

Cadmium is a toxic substance that is found in pesticides and enamel coating. It reaches human beings by means of vegetables and grains, mainly, as well as water that has been softened by chemicals, or molluscs and oysters.

Cadmium is considered more toxic than lead, and is found in cigarette smoke, in nickel-cadmium batteries, and in processed coffee products (such as decaffeinated coffee).

The signs of cadmium toxicity include: atherosclerosis, emphysema, and chronic bronchitis; high blood pressure; lung and kidney problems to the point of cancer; heart diseases and problems; and anemia due to a shortage of iron. You can protect yourself against cadmium toxicity by eating foods that are rich in zinc (such as pumpkin seeds, nuts, and so on), because zinc is a cadmium antagonist; taking vitamin C, which is the specific defense; by avoiding using utensils with enamel coatings (use glass or stainless steel utensils instead); by avoiding white flour products from which the zinc has been extracted (during the whitening process), and only the cadmium remains; if possible, by drinking filtered water or mineral/natural water, and not water from the faucet; by decreasing your consumption of coffee and tea, as cadmium is found in both of them, and by totally avoiding decaffeinated coffee!

Calcium

Chemical symbol Ca, specific gravity 1.55, atomic weight 40.01 (calcium).

Calcium is a metallic chemical element found in our bodies, and one of the most widespread in nature (limestone and chalk are made of calcium). It is gray in color, and creates various compounds easily both in the body and in nature (and in various industries). Calcium is the most important substance for the building of the skeleton and bones: 99% is found in the bones and teeth, and 1% in the soft tissues. It is of enormous importance in the muscles and the heart muscle.

Together with magnesium, calcium regulates the heart rate, and also completes the action of other minerals in the digestive system. Every year, the body "recycles" 20% (one-fifth) of the amount of calcium by releasing calcium from the tissues and the bones and replenishing it from food.

This continuous action does not only occur during menopause, but all our lives, and when our nutrition is poor in (organic) calcium, which must be absorbed back into the bones (which are the reserves of calcium), cumulative damage is caused over the years to the walls of the bones and to the bone itself, which becomes absorbed - and suddenly people become aware of a process that is called "calcium loss."

The shortage of calcium can also be caused (and this is the process that occurs generally) when food is rich in phosphorus (too rich, in relation to calcium), and when the diet consists of meat (beef, chicken, and so on), in which the proportion of phosphorus to calcium is opposite to that in human beings - 40 times more!

It is important to know that menopausal vegetarian women lose only 18% of their bone mass, while menopausal carnivorous women lose over 35% - and that is in addition to the loss of calcium over the years prior to menopause.

In order for calcium to be absorbed in the stomach, normal stomach acid (hydrochloride - HCl) is required, as is vitamin D. Its absorption is easier when it comes from unpasteurized dairy products.

The mechanism in a healthy person's stomach contains a "safety" device that prevents the absorption of excessive calcium in the blood, and allows the excess (including the excess from supplements) to pass through harmlessly. When the safety mechanism is defective and there is excessive calcium, problems of calcinosis and hypercalcemia are liable to occur.

In order for calcium to be absorbed in the body and to function properly, calcium - and our bodies - needs magnesium, phosphorus, vitamins A, C, and D, and good proteins.

Absorption occurs mainly in the duodenum (in a short time and at a length of 12 inches only).

Calcium problems are likely when the parathyroid hormone is secreted incorrectly, and then an excess of calcium is revealed in blood tests, meaning that calcium is coming out of the bones. This condition must be treated thoroughly.

Calcium influences the action and stimulation of the muscles, and balances potassium and sodium in muscle tension. It is needed for regulating the heart rate, and for the blood coagulation mechanism. Calcium is necessary for transmitting nervous information via nervous impulses, and for activating the hormones that are linked to metabolism. It is important in the metabolism of iron. Calcium safeguards bones and teeth. It is of cardinal importance for the growth of children's bones in general, and for adolescents going through growth spurts. It alleviates growing pains, as well as insomnia.

The recommended dietary allowance of calcium is as follows: for infants of up to 6 months, it is 360 mg, for infants of between 6 and 12 months, it is 540 mg, for children of up to 10 years, it is 800 mg, for youngsters of between 11 and 18 years, it is 1,000 mg, for people over 18 years, it is 800 mg. Pregnant and nursing women should add 400 mg.

People who suffer from backaches, joint problems, difficult menstrual periods, hypoglycemia (lack of sugar), and high blood pressure should take higher doses - under medical supervision, of course.

Calcium is found in the following foods: all dried herbs, almonds, green leafy vegetables - mainly broccoli and parsley, dried brewer's yeast, filberts, soy flour, dairy products from goats, sheep, and cows, small fish (in the bones), peanuts, soy, dried legumes, sesame paste, and sunflower seeds. Smaller amounts are found in all fruits and vegetables.

If there is a shortage of calcium, the following symptoms are liable to occur: calcium loss - osteoporosis; delayed growth in children; menstrual problems, including lengthy periods/heavy bleeding; nervousness, irritation, poor sleep; poor quality and shape of bones and teeth, leading to leg cramps - tetany; rickets and osteomalacia.

There is toxicity in calcium in daily doses of over 2,000 mg, and with a problematic stomach, there could be a problem of excess - hypercalcemia. This does not include therapeutic cases, in which there is a definite need for more calcium, such as arthritis (and as I mentioned earlier, also in a case where the thyroid gland creates the problem.)

Supplements for calcium are available in the following forms: calcium + magnesium made from dolomite rock; calcium with vitamins to help its absorption; calcium + magnesium, at a proportion of 2:1; calcium + magnesium + boron; and bone meal tablets.

Calcium should be of the lactate type, which originates in milk; or, alternatively, of the gluconate type, which is of plant origin - it is preferable, and is better absorbed in the body.

Chlorine

Chemical symbol Cl, atomic weight 35.46 (chlorum).

Chlorine is a non-metal gas, from the halogen group (chlorine, fluorine, bromide, and iodine). Its color is greenish - hence its name, which comes from the Greek chloros - "pale green."It has a pungent odor, and is found in nature in compounds of cooking salt (sodium chloride).

Chlorine is used as a bleach and a disinfectant. It is a mineral that is necessary for nutrition, and serves as an important component in the stomach acid (hydrochloride).

If large quantities are added to the water in swimming pools, children's (and adults') teeth are liable to be destroyed, and the same thing is liable to happen when drinking water has been chlorinated in order to purify it. You should always boil chlorinated water or let it stand for a few hours until the chlorine (which is a gas) evaporates.

Chlorine regulates the acid-base balance in the blood. It works with sodium and potassium as a compound, and helps clean the body by helping the liver's action. It maintains the body's pliancy and muscle tone, and helps convey and distribute the hormones throughout the body. Since it is a component of the stomach acid, it is helpful in digestion, especially of proteins.

The daily recommended dietary allowance for infants up to 6 months is 0.275-0.7 g, for infants of 6 to 12 months is 0.4-1.2 g, for children of 1-3 years is 0.5-1.5 g, for children of 4-6 years is 0.7-2.1 g, for children of 7-10 years is 0.925-2.775 g, for youngsters of 11-17 years is 1.4-4.2 g, and for people over 18 years is 1.75-5.1 g. It should be noted that in regular nutrition, there is enough salt, which means that there is a regular supply of chlorine, and sometimes even an excess.

Chlorine can be found in the following foods: salt (cooking or sea), seaweed, vegetables (root vegetables contain sodium chloride, leafy vegetables contain potassium chloride), and olives.

People who suffer from high blood pressure (which conventional medicine calls “from an unknown source”) are advised to avoid salt and salty foods.

A shortage of chlorine is very rare, unless there is vomiting and/or diarrhea, which expels it, and then it cannot perform its functions. If there is a shortage, it could result in hair and teeth loss.

Chlorine has no toxicity, but daily consumption in excess of 14 g can cause disturbances in the body and lead to unpleasant and toxic side-effects. Even a smaller amount than this can damage the intestinal flora, and impair the production of vitamin B. It may not be toxic, but in large quantities, chlorine disrupts the production of thyroxine, thus weakening the immune system, not to mention that chlorine leads to arteriosclerosis and heart diseases.

Chromium

Chemical symbol Cr, specific gravity 6.7, atomic weight 52.01 (chromium).

Chromium is a hard metal that shines when polished. It is bluish-white in color, and its name derives from the Greek word chroma, meaning "color." It is used in the steel industry. Chromium salts are used in the paint, glass, and tanning industries. Chromium is destroyed during the processing of food, and experimental attempts have been made to reintroduce it into food in order to avoid atherosclerosis - a scientific fact that has been proved beyond a shadow of a doubt.

Research has shown that the problem of diabetes is directly linked to nutrition and to a shortage of chromium in the modern diet. Chromium is linked to the regulation of insulin production in the pancreas, and increases its efficiency, so that when there is a shortage of chromium, the pancreas produces low-grade insulin (and a lot of it), thus creating a totally useless strain on the pancreas until its action slows down and finally halts.

The amount of chromium in the body decreases with age, and an interesting phenomenon has been discovered: new-born infants and babies consume a great deal of chromium during pregnancy, which causes their mothers' chromium supply to dwindle.

This action does not occur in primitive populations, whose chromium level remains stable in their bodies even during old age - and this is not surprising, since their food is not processed (that is, until "progress" catches up with them).

Chromium always acts in conjunction with other organic factors: with iron, it carries proteins in the blood, and with certain organic links, it is active in the metabolism of sugar; it is called Chromium GTF (glucose tolerant factor) when its activity is not only in the context of diabetes, but also in that of hypoglycemia.

Chromium increases the effectiveness of insulin (both natural and external). It balances the sugars in the body for both diabetes and hypoglycemia. It lowers the levels of cholesterol and fats in the blood, and treats atherosclerosis. It lowers high blood pressure, and helps in growth (in children).

While there are no recommended dietary allowances, the daily amount required for infants of up to 6 months is 0.01-0.04 mg, for children of 6-12 months is 0.02-0.06 mg, for children of 1-3 years is 0.02-0.08 mg, for children of 4-6 years is 0.03-0.12 mg, and for people of 7 and over is 0.05-0.20 mg.

Sometimes, when there is a need for chromium (something that is revealed in hair tests, which show shortages or excesses of minerals and vitamins), it is customary to administer zinc (either alone, or with a chromium supplement), and this improves the chromium situation and the absorption of chromium. A therapeutic dose is much higher than a normal daily amount, and is prescribed by a physician.

Natural chromium tablets, which are suitable for this, are available, as are pure chromium tablets and chromium + selenium tablets. Generally speaking, a sufficient quantity of chromium is found in natural multivitamin and multimineral tablets. People who take brewer's yeast tablets (not torula yeast) obtain chromium from the tablets.

Chromium can be found in the following foods: whole wheat, brown rice, and other whole grains, whole oatmeal porridge, legumes, nuts, dried brewer's yeast, corn oil, meat, and chicken. Fruit and vegetables contain very little chromium.

If there is a shortage of chromium, the following diseases and conditions may occur: diabetes or hypoglycemia, arteriosclerosis, cholesterol/fats and/or heart problems, or even low cholesterol. Remember that a shortage of chromium is linked to a diet of processed food.

Chromium has no known toxicity. Having said that, it must be pointed out that an especially large daily amount of chromium is liable to cause nausea.

Cobalt

Chemical symbol Co, specific gravity 8.90, atomic weight 58.94 (cobaltum).

Cobalt is an extremely heavy metal, similar in color to steel. It is used in the manufacture of especially hard metal tools. Its dark blue color and name are derived from the German word Kobold (devil's child), since the German miners thought that it had diabolical and harmful properties.

Cobalt-60 is a radioactive isotope of cobalt, and is used mainly for treating cancerous tissues during radiation therapy. Cobalt is an essential mineral, and it is part of vitamin B12, which is also called cyanocobalamin. It comes mainly from animals, as well as from marine vegetation.

Cobalt is needed for the production of red blood cells, and for the enzymatic system.

Cobalt does not have any toxicity, and there are no daily recommended dietary allowances for it. However, excessive cobalt causes problems in the thyroid gland, something which is extremely rare.

If there is a shortage of cobalt, the phenomena that may occur are identical to those that occur with a shortage of iron or vitamin B12.

Copper

Chemical symbol Cu, specific gravity 8.92, atomic weight 63.57 (cuprum).

Copper is a trace element that is essential for the body, and is found in every cell. It is a soft, reddish-yellow metal that is an excellent conductor of electricity. It is used in the tool industry, especially in the form of bronze or brass.

In the body, it is consumed in milligrams. While the body absolutely cannot be without it, over-consumption is forbidden. Not much is known about copper, but there are many differences of opinion because of the difficulty in investigating it, so I will outline the things that are known for sure.

Copper serves as one of the components that cover, strengthen and insulate the nerve walls with vitamin B (and especially folic acid). It is necessary for the absorption of iron, and essential for its absorption in the blood and its conversion into hemoglobin. Copper is linked to the (positive) oxidation of vitamin C, and to the building of RNA, as well as to the metabolism of proteins. It is necessary for the strengthening of the bones. It is linked to the pigments in the skin and hair (with the amino acid tyrosine.)

There is no daily recommended dietary allowance for copper. The estimated safe daily intake is as follows: for infants up to 6 months, it is 0.5-0.7 mg, for infants of between 6 and 12 months, it is 0.7-1.0 mg, for children of between 1 and 3 years, it is 1.0-1.5 mg, for children of between 4 and 6 years, it is 1.5-2.0 mg, for children of between 7 and 10 years, it is 2.0-2.5 mg, and for people of 11 years and over, it is 2.0-3.0 mg.

The amount of copper should be increased if there is a consumption of zinc: for every extra 50 mg of zinc, 2 mg of copper should be added, since these two minerals "compete" with each other, but both are necessary.

Copper is found in the following foods: whole grains (whole wheat, brown rice, and so on), buckwheat, dried brewer's yeast, molasses, mushrooms, walnuts, lentils, and green leafy vegetables.

Copper is not destroyed easily, and correct nutrition is sufficient to ensure the right amount of it.

If there is a shortage of copper, the following symptoms may occur: calcium loss, anemia, and general weakness; respiratory problems and edemas; nervous disorders (because of the damage to the myelin - the nerve covering); sores on the skin, and hair loss.

Copper toxicity is extremely rare, unless it is taken in enormous quantities. Unnecessary copper supplements occur in places where there are copper water pipes, and copper cooking utensils are used.

In most cases, copper is found in multimineral and multivitamin formulas or tablets, and there is hardly any need to take it separately (except in a therapeutic situation, under medical supervision).

Excess copper has been found in people who suffer from mental depression.

Fluorine

Chemical symbol F, specific gravity 1.69, atomic weight 9 (fluorine).

Fluorine is a mineral that is found in every tissue in the body. It is essential especially for bones and teeth, in that it helps calcium to be absorbed in the necessary places. Excessive fluorine is toxic (to the point of death), and when it is found in water at a proportion of more than 2 parts per million, it harms the teeth, causing them to appear spotty.

Fluorine is found in two forms:

Calcium fluoride - its natural form (and the one that is necessary for the body).

Sodium fluoride - its synthetic (and toxic) form, whose addition to drinking water is highly controversial.

The gigantic metal companies are guilty of lobbying for the use of synthetic fluoride (which is a by-product of the steel industry), because in this way, they spare themselves the bother of having to find a place to store it.

Fluoride must not be taken as a supplement, unless prescribed by a physician, and even then, it must be used in its natural form.

An amount of over 20 mg a day is toxic.

If there is a shortage of fluorine, there can be problems and weakness in the bones and teeth. If there is an excess (toxicity) of fluorine, the following symptoms may occur: problems and weakness in the teeth (spotty teeth); the destruction of phosphatase, which is the enzyme that is important in the metabolism of vitamins; damage to the brain tissue - in places where the water is rich in fluoride, there is an increase in the percentage of children with

Down's syndrome; damage to the bones - research has shown that people who live in areas where the water is rich in fluorides (fluorinated water, to which fluorine has been added), there is a higher percentage of bone fractures in the elderly.

In this case, calcium protects against the toxicity of fluorine.

Iodine

Chemical symbol I, atomic weight 126.9 (iodum).

Iodine is a non-metal, chemical element from the halogen group (chlorine, fluorine, bromide, and iodine). Its color is deep purple, and hence its name, which comes from the word ioeides - "violet-colored" in Greek. Every body needs iodine. Iodine salts are used in the photographic industry and in medicine.

The general amount that is found in our body is about 10-25 mg, and most of it is in the thyroid gland. This means that a minor shortage of iodine can cause problems in the thyroid gland (which is found in the front part of the throat), leading to problems with metabolism in the cells of the tissues, with the regulation of digestion, and with the regulation of heat in the body. A slowing-down of metabolism (in the activity of the thyroid gland) results in a slowing-down of or decrease in hormone production, sensitivity to cold, fatigue and drowsiness, apathy, and weight-gain, since iodine constitutes an integral part of the hormone thyroxine, which is the principal hormone of the thyroid gland, and it has additional actions: converting carotene into vitamin A, absorption of carbohydrates in the small intestine, and the digestion and burning of fats.

In the form of a medication, iodine can be dangerous, but there is no risk when it appears in food. There are foods that contain anti-thyroxine substances, and decrease the action of iodine, such as the cabbage family (if eaten in large quantities) and mustard seeds.

Iodine prevents the rise of blood-fats, and arterio-sclerosis. Furthermore, it promotes correct growth, improves learning, and enhances and accelerates thought processes (mental agility). It improves general energy, and controls and balances weight (by burning excess fat) - and for this reason is good for dieting. Iodine is helpful for the growth and maintenance of healthy hair, nails, teeth, and skin.

The daily recommended dietary allowance for infants up to the age of 6 months is 40 mcg, for infants up to the age of 1 year is 50 mcg, for children of between 1 and 3 years is 70 mcg, for children of between 4 and 6 years is 90 mcg, for children of between 7 and 10 years is 120 mcg, and for people of 11 onward is 150 mcg. Pregnant women should take 25 mcg more, and nursing women should take 50 mcg more. Therapeutic doses are higher - sometimes six or ten times higher - but only under medical supervision.

Iodine is found in the following foods: seaweed (fresh or in tablet form), marine fish, sea food, vegetables, and onions grown in iodine-rich soil

The major part of iodine supplement during the therapeutic period (such as during a diet for losing weight) will be in the form of seaweed tablets, or from cooking seaweed and drinking it.

If there is a shortage of iodine, the following symptoms may occur: goiter, a disease of the thyroid gland; weight-gain, or alternatively difficulty in losing weight; psychological and mental disturbances; impaired release of energy, leading to sluggishness; a lower body temperature, which can indicate hypo-activity (under-activity) of the thyroid gland; and lastly, coarse, dry skin.

Comment: Sometimes, when there is a shortage of iodine (not even a serious shortage), there is a slowing-down of the action of the thyroid gland. Even if blood tests apparently show that the hormone level is normal (within the parameters), we know from experience that in almost everyone whose weight is higher than normal, his/her thyroid gland is working too slowly (too slowly in relation to his/her weight).

The only time there is toxicity in iodine is when synthetic iodine supplements are taken (as medications). There is no toxicity in natural supplements to food, but in very large quantities, hyperactivity and nervousness can occur. Sometimes there are people who are allergic to iodine, and most of them have a history of a use of medical iodine for tests and X-rays.

Iron

Chemical symbol Fe, specific gravity 7.87, atomic weight 55.8 (ferrum).

Iron is a chemical element. It is the metal that has been most commonly used for thousands of years, and is (almost) not found in nature in its pure form.

Iron is a mineral that is necessary for life, and it belongs to the group of minerals that must be consumed in small quantities. (Just to remind you - the second group must be consumed in large quantities, including magnesium and calcium.)

More than half of the iron in the body is used as a compound in the red blood cells (hemoglobin) together with protein and copper, and it also participates in the creation of myoglobin, which is the protein that stores oxygen in the muscle (in the red color).

Iron is found in every cell in the body. For its assimilation in the body (and its transport) vitamin C, folic acid, vitamin E, copper, manganese, and cobalt are required, and there must be a balance with calcium and phosphorus and with the rest of the vitamin B complex. For its absorption, the presence of hydrochloric acid (HCl) in the stomach is necessary, and a digestive protein that regulates its absorption via the mucous membranes.

Iron and calcium constitute the primary nutrient deficiencies in women, and in order not to reach the point of deficiency, nutrients for several basic processes must be provided. Remember that during a single month, women lose double the amount of iron that men do.

Iron renews itself in the body naturally, and red blood

cells renew themselves every four months (120 days). For this to occur, there must be balance, as I mentioned above.

There are several points to remember about iron:

Its absorption in the body is less than 5%; therefore, during the course of a day, an amount no smaller than 400 mg of iron (organic) must be consumed in order for the required amount to be absorbed.

Drinking regular tea reduces the absorption of iron by between a third and a half because of the tannic acid in it, and drinking coffee after a meal reduces the absorption of iron by more than a third.

Preservatives and anti-oxidants in food, such as BHTA, phosphatase, or EDTA, prevent the absorption of iron (as well as the rest of the minerals, especially zinc and magnesium).

When there is a need for iron supplements (in tablet form) for people who suffer from anemia or low hemoglobin, or for pregnant women, they must demand organic iron whose absorption and assimilation are better than the ferrous sulfate (which is not organic) that is supplied by the drug companies (mainly), and sometimes also cause constipation and nausea, and damage the vitamin E in the body.

In pernicious anemia, iron with the addition of B complex and especially B12 is needed. In leukemia or colitis, iron is needed, and it must be remembered that with problems such as cirrhosis of the liver and diabetes (that derives from impaired functioning of the pancreas), iron deposits can form as a result of taking excessive doses. In cases of sickle-cell anemia or hemochromatosis or thalassemia, iron must not be taken in a concentrated form, and sometimes another mineral (such as zinc) is required in order to treat the problem.

The roles of iron include: curing and preventing anemia, increasing energy by reducing fatigue, improving the color of the blood (and the color of children's cheeks), helping growth in children, improving resistance to disease, and improving the transport of oxygen in the blood to the cells.

The recommended dietary allowance of iron for infants up to 6 months is 10 mg, for children of between 6 months and 3 years is 15 mg, for children of between 4 and 10 years is 10 mg, for males of between 11 and 18 years is 18 mg, and for adult males is 10 mg. For females of between 11 and 50, the amount is 18 mg; above 50, it is 10 mg. Pregnant and lactating women should add between 30 and 60 mg.

Iron can be found in the following foods: dried vegetables and herbs, dried brewer's yeast, whole sesame seed and whole sesame paste, molasses, soy flour, dried legumes (chickpeas, fava beans, lentils, black-eyed peas), fish, cashew nuts, pine nuts, almonds, peanuts, calf liver (be careful of hormones and antibiotics), meat (the inner organs), green leafy vegetables, and chicken.

Meat: You should eat "organic" meat, that is, meat that does not contain hormones and antibiotics, substances that cause damage to the human body, such as hormonal upsets, especially in women.

The amount of iron in (natural) multivitamin tablets is sufficient for the daily requirement, but not for therapeutic purposes.

If there is a shortage of iron, the following symptoms may occur: anemia, a shortage of red blood cells, a low rate of red-blood-cell formation, a decline in the blood supply to the cells, especially to the muscles, depression and lack of appetite, a slowing down of cerebral activity (impaired memory), weakness, vertigo, pallor, hair loss, and shortness of breath.

Toxicity is rare, unless iron is taken during illnesses (as I listed before), or a daily dosage of over 100 mg is taken over an extended period.

It must be remembered that non-organic iron is supplied in amounts larger than 100 mg in the knowledge that only 10% of it will be absorbed in the body, and for this reason, it is preferable to consume only natural iron.

Lead

Chemical symbol Pb, specific gravity 11.34, atomic weight 20.721 (plumbum).

Lead is a soft, rust-resistant metal that is used for pipes, soldering, and casting (of characters in printing).

If lead reaches the bone, it replaces the calcium; for this reason, calcium-rich food will help in avoiding the absorption of lead.

Lead poisoning is becoming an ecological disease that is developing very rapidly. In addition to exhaust fumes that are rich in lead, people absorb lead from smoking and passive smoking. Lead poisoning can be fatal to human beings, even in small quantities, which is why gasoline is now sold in an unleaded form. Moreover, lead is being removed from commercial paints and children's paints, from ceramics, and so on. Lead and its toxicity accumulate in the body, and, as can be seen from the list of symptoms, it is difficult to identify lead poisoning as the cause.

The signs of lead poisoning include: multiple sclerosis - neuro-muscular diseases; stomach-aches, vertigo, and headaches; hyperactivity in children; anemia, nervousness, fatigue, and loss of appetite; damage to the liver, kidneys, and heart; partial paralysis of the limbs; blindness and mental disturbances (from the accumulation of lead in the head); problems in the reproductive system (and impotence in men); and impaired growth in infants and children whose mothers suffered from lead poisoning;.

You can protect yourself from lead poisoning by consuming the following: calcium, vitamin D (in combination with calcium); vitamin C in therapeutic daily doses of at least 1,000-3,000 mg; vitamin B1, which is especially valuable for this; at least 25,000 International Units of vitamin A; lecithin, potassium iodide that binds to the lead in the body and helps to excrete it; legumes, beans, and algin from seaweed (in powder form).

Magnesium

Chemical symbol Mg, specific gravity 1.74, atomic weight 24.3 (magnesium).

Magnesium is a light metallic, chemical element that burns with a very strong light. Its color is white (silver). In industry, it is combined with aluminum, and it is used in the aircraft industry and in medicine.

Magnesium is one of the most important minerals in the human body, and it operates with and complements calcium in the building of bones and muscles. Magnesium is found in nerve fluids, and causes muscle fibers to release tension, while calcium stimulates the muscle fibers to contract. This action also occurs in the heart, which is a muscle. The calcium contracts the muscle, and the magnesium contributes to its release and regulates the heartbeat.

Both magnesium and calcium constitute a component in the gums. Only in recent years has magnesium been "acknowledged" by the medical establishment (while in homeopathic medicine, it has been known as a positive factor for years). The total amount of magnesium in the body is slightly more than 20 grams, and it is a mineral that helps the body under conditions of stress. Research has revealed that children who suffer from convulsions and nervous disorders must take more magnesium, and milk must be omitted from their diets, because the fluorides in milk bind to the magnesium and remove it. People who eat refined or processed foods (such as refined carbohydrates or alcohol) must increase their magnesium intake, as must people who take diuretics, or women who take oral contraceptives. Low quantities of magnesium in the body lead to destructive diseases (including cancer).

Magnesium is an antacid and counteracts the stomach acid, so it should not be taken with or soon after a meal containing protein (that requires stomach acid), or early in the morning.

Magnesium is necessary for the absorption of calcium and the assimilation of vitamin C, as well as for the conversion of blood sugar into energy. It activates enzymatic systems that require various biological actions, and is essential for maintaining RNA/DNA. It is necessary for the synthesis of several amino acids, as well as for dissolving kidney stones (with vitamin B6), and for the normal contraction of the muscles. Magnesium also gets rid of body odor and halitosis (as do zinc, vitamin B6 and PABA). It is important for maintaining the health of the gums, and is necessary for the regulation of body fluids (swelling in the face, joints, etc.), and for regulating the heartbeat rate. Magnesium alleviates heartburn (as an antacid), digestive problems and pains, and helps to combat depression.

The daily recommended dietary allowance of magnesium for infants up to 6 months old is 50 mg, for infants of between 6 and 12 months is 70 mg, for children of between 1 and 3 years is 150 mg, for children of between 4 and 6 years is 200 mg, for children of between 7 and 10 years is 250 mg. For males of between 11 and 14 years, the RDA is 350 mg, for males of between 15 and 18 years it is 400 mg, and over that age is 350 mg. For females of over 11 years, the RDA is 300 mg, while pregnant and nursing women should take an additional 150 mg (under medical supervision, of course).

Children whose diet contains a lot of protein must increase their intake, and those who consume milk must increase their intake of magnesium-rich food. Adults who consume alcohol, milk and dairy products, and proteins must increase their magnesium intake.

Magnesium is found in the following foods: most fruits and vegetables such as figs, citrus fruit, apples (especially dark green ones), in dried herbs, soy flour, nuts, almonds, molasses, brewer's yeast, buckwheat, legumes (especially black-eyed peas), whole wheat, brown rice, oatmeal, cornstarch, dried onions, and millet.

Magnesium is present in natural tablets that are combined with vitamin B6, as well as in natural tablets/chealates or combined with calcium (at a proportion of 1:2) or combined with calcium + boron.

If there is a shortage of magnesium, the following symptoms may occur: atherosclerosis, high blood pressure, irregular heartbeat, calcium stones - especially in people whose consumption of dairy products is high, over-stimulation of muscles and nerves, nervous tics and contractions, convulsions, and fits.

There is toxicity only when taken in very large doses over a long time. A daily dosage of 30 grams or more has been found to be harmful.

The body absorbs only about a third of the amount of magnesium that it consumes, so that no less than 120 mg must be taken in order to ensure the minimal amount (this is much less than a harmful amount).

Manganese

Chemical symbol Mn, specific gravity 7.3, atomic weight 54.93 (manganium).

Manganese is a hard, brittle element. It has a silvery color, and is used in combination with iron in order to obtain superior steel. In the lighting industry, it is used for yellow lighting. In the body, its action is complex, which makes research about it difficult. In recent years, additional information pertaining to manganese has emerged, but since there are still no medications for problems caused by a shortage of manganese, no conclusions have been reached yet.

The body secretes 4-5 mg of manganese every day, which is the minimal daily amount. It has been found that a larger quantity of manganese is required for meat-eaters and consumers of dairy products, since the exaggerated amounts of calcium and phosphorus impair the absorption of manganese.

Manganese helps the pancreas in its function and in the correct use of glucose. It serves as a component of the bones (as a collagen supplement), as well as the glue that binds calcium, magnesium, and phosphorus. It is active in the production of thyroxine (the thyroid gland's hormone), and sex hormones. It is important in the production of cholesterol and in the breakdown and composition of fats. It strengthens the bone cartilage, as well as the points where the muscles are joined to the bones. It serves as a component in the nervous system (a neurotransmitter, acetylcholine). It plays a role in the enzymes for the absorption of vitamin B_1, biotin, vitamin C, and choline, as well as in the prevention of sterility. With lecithin, it improves the memory and concentration, and reduces stress.

No daily recommended dietary allowance has been established. The estimated safe daily intake is as follows: For infants of up to 6 months, it is 0.5-0.7 mg, for infants of between 7 and 12 months, it is 0.7-1.0 mg, for children of between 1 and 3 years, it is 1.0-1.5 mg, for children of between 4 and 6 years, it is 1.5-2.0 mg, for children of between 7 and 10 years, it is 2.0-3.0 mg, and for people over 11 years, it is 2.5-5.0 mg.

If large amounts of dairy products and meat are consumed, larger quantities of manganese are required.

Manganese is contained in natural multimineral and multivitamin tablets and formulas.

Manganese is found in the following foods: mainly in whole grains (brown rice, whole wheat, etc,), egg yolks, walnuts, almonds, peanuts, green leafy vegetables, peas, beets, avocado, barley, whole oats, and in most vegetables and fruits (that have not undergone industrial processes).

If there is a shortage of manganese, the following symptoms may occur: multiple sclerosis, soft bones, weakness in ligaments and tendons; weakness in the muscles (a lack of muscular coordination - ataxia or myasthenia gravis - serious muscle weakness); disrupted nerve actions and mental confusion; sexual indifference; recurring vertigo; digestive disorders, and impaired metabolism (connected to the thyroid gland); an increase in blood sugar; slow growth and development.

Manganese toxicity is extremely rare, and is liable to be created by industrial toxins. As a rule, there is no need to take too much of it.

Mercury

Chemical symbol Hg, specific gravity 14.2, atomic weight 200.6 (hydrargyrum).

Mercury is a heavy metallic chemical element that is found in nature in a liquid form (at a normal temperature). The color of mercury resembles that of silver, and it is used in thermometers and other scientific instruments. As a chemical compound in nitric acid and alcohol, it is used for filling detonators, fuses, and mercury-detonated bullets.

Mercury is poisonous to human beings, and as a result of the dumping of industrial waste, it is found in lakes and rivers in the form of a substance called methyl-mercury, and that it how it gets into fishes and from there into people.

Fungicidal sprays for foodstuffs contain mercury, and this is another way in which mercury gets into the human body. There are also medications that contain mercury chloride, which contributes to the accumulation of mercury in the body.

Signs of hydrargyrism (mercury poisoning) include: damage to the brain and the central nervous system; disturbances of enzymatic actions in the body; damage to the kidneys and liver, to the point of blindness and paralyses; tremors, mental degeneration, diarrhea, and speech difficulties.

In order to defend ourselves against mercury, the following are recommended: dried brewer's yeast, since it contains selenium (see "Selenium"); calcium, since it neutralizes almost all poisons (see "Calcium"); lecithin and hydrochloride; taking vitamins from the anti-oxidant group on a daily basis (A, B, C, E); refraining from eating food that has been sprayed with insecticides, and from drinking unfiltered water from the faucet.

Molybdenum

Chemical symbol Mo, specific gravity 0.2, atomic weight 42 (molybdenum).

There is very little information about the trace mineral molybdenum. It is a component of several enzymes, and it is linked to the production of red blood cells, as well as to the metabolism of fats and carbohydrates.

Molybdenum helps to extract the iron from its storage places in the liver, and is active in fighting anemia. It promotes a general feeling of good health. It has an effect that prevents tooth decay.

There is no daily recommended dietary allowance for molybdenum, but the estimated safe daily intake is as follows: For infants of up to 6 months, it is 0.03-0.06 mg, for infants of between 6 and 12 months, it is 0.04-0.06 mg, for children of between 1 and 3 years, it is 0.05-0.10 mg, for children of between 4 and 6 years, it is 0.06-0.15 mg, for children of between 7 and 10 years, it is 0.10-0.30 mg, and for people of 11 years and over, it is 0.15-0.50 mg.

Molybdenum is contained in most natural multivitamin and multimineral formulas.

Molybdenum is found in the following foods: whole grains, dark vegetables, and legumes. The molybdenum content depends on the quality of the soil.

The symptoms of a shortage of molybdenum are unknown.

Molybdenum's toxicity is unknown, but huge quantities are liable to cause a shortage of copper, something that is extremely rare. Special attention should be paid to molybdenum only in cases of the entire diet consisting of processed food, and completely lacking in nutritional value.

Nickel

Chemical symbol Ni, specific gravity 8.90, atomic weight 58.69 (nickel).

Nickel is a hard, white, shiny metal that does not rust, and it is therefore used in the production process of metals and steel. Its name is derived from the German word Kupfer-nickel.

Nickel's main functions have not yet been finally clarified, even though we know that it activates a number of enzymatic systems in the body, and is found in high concentrations in RNA.

This is one of the groups of trace metals that is necessary for us in small amounts, and since it is found in mainly in vegetables, it is not problematic. Apparently, it is not necessary as a separate supplement.

Nickel toxicity occurs only through industrial poisons.

There are no nickel supplements, and it is not contained in vitamin or mineral tablets, since its main functions have not yet been defined, and the required amount seems to be found in food.

Phosphorus

Chemical symbol P, atomic weight 13 (phosphorus).

Phosphorus is common in a compound form in nature, since it is found in every living cell.

The mineral is found in two forms: the white form that is highly flammable, hence the name phos, which means "light," and phor, which means "carrier" (in Greek); and the red form, which is stable.

The phosphorus compounds are phosphates - chemical fertilizers.

Phosphorus operates together with calcium. In the bones, there is more calcium and less phosphorus, and in the soft tissues, the opposite is true. Phosphorus is involved with and linked to the chemical actions of all the cells.

Phosphorus is important for the absorption of vitamins B2 and B3, and it plays a part in the metabolism of carbohydrates and fats. Moreover, it is significant for growth and heredity. It is an important component of phospholipids (such as lecithin), which are crucial for the breakdown of fats and the cholesterol balance, and it is also important for normal hormonal secretion.

Pregnant women are advised to take more phosphorus than normal, and in the proportion of phosphorus to calcium (1 phosphorus to 25 calcium), it must be remembered that children need more calcium, and care must be taken not to upset the balance.

There is a direct link between the consumption of phosphorus (from food) and the state of the bones and calcium loss, and that is because meat contains 40 times more phosphorus than calcium!

University studies that have investigated osteoporosis have found that in women who are vegetarians (and consume eggs and dairy products), calcium loss is only about half of what it is in carnivorous women, who lose calcium from the bones to the tune of 35%, and this loss weakens the bones. The processed food industry uses phosphorus (mainly in the form of a compound with sodium), which causes the amount of phosphorus that is consumed by the body to be higher than what it should be.

For instance, baking powder contains phosphorus and sodium salt, which gives flour a whiter color. (Phosphorus and calcium salt is more balanced.) Preservatives are connected to phosphoric acid in that those kinds of compounds make it difficult for bacteria to reproduce. Phosphorus salt is added to raw meat that is not fresh (or to salty cheeses) in order to disguise the unpleasant odor.

Another example is soft drinks, which, in addition to food colorings, also include phosphorus, giving them a slightly sour taste, and also increasing the life-span of the bubbles of gas. However, it washes away the calcium in the digestive system, and prevents the absorption of magnesium in the blood by means of a compound that is not absorbable. The study that revealed these facts also showed that damage is caused to the zinc balance.

The salt imbalance that is caused by eating processed foods (white and nice-looking) and drinking soft drinks destroys every healthy part,, and for this reason, you should read labels to see if phosphorus appears as sodium phosphate, calcium phosphate or sodium pyrophosphate.

Phosphorus accelerates the healing of bone fractures, and other fractures and damage. It promotes growth, and contributes to the strengthening of teeth and gums. It reduces the pains of arthritis, and increases the energy for studying and athletic activity by means of the metabolism of fats and carbohydrates. Phosphorus is a component of myelin - the substance that constitutes the nerve sheaths that transmit nervous impulses. It halts the level of acidity in the body.

It should be noted that aluminum and excessive iron and magnesium render phosphorus ineffective.

The daily recommended amount for infants up to 2 months is 240-500 mg, for infants up to 1 year is 360-500 mg, for children up to 3 years is 500-800 mg, for children up to 10 years is 800-1,000 mg, and for youngsters up to 18 years is 1,000-1,200 mg. The daily recommended dietary allowance for adults is 800-1,200 mg, with the higher amount recommended for pregnant or nursing women.

Phosphorus can be found in the following foods: fish, chicken, beef, eggs, whole grains, nuts, sunflower seeds, pumpkin seeds, and sesame seeds. Remember that the foods that are richer in phosphorus than they are in calcium (besides the various kinds of meat) are: avocado, nuts and almonds, eggs, sunflower seeds, bananas, lecithin, wheat-germ and bran, soy, brewer's yeast, legumes, lentils, and mushrooms.

It is highly recommended - especially after age 40 - to cut down on the consumption of all kinds of meat, and to increase the amount of green leafy vegetables, since after this age, there are problems with the absorption of excess phosphorus by the kidneys.

If there is a shortage of phosphorus, the following symptoms may occur: weak bones and teeth (weakness in the gums), rickets, arthritis, respiratory problems, fatigue (including mental fatigue), and pus in the body and in the gums.

Phosphorus is not known to be toxic, but excessive amounts of it harm other balances, as was explained above (especially calcium).

Potassium

Chemical symbol K (not to be confused with vitamin K), specific gravity 0.86, atomic weight 39.096 (kalium).

Potassium is a metal that is not found freely in nature, but rather in various compounds. Potassium works in conjunction with sodium for the balance and regulation of the body's fluids, since potassium is found in most of the fluids in the cells (the intracellular fluid), and the major amount of sodium is found in the intercellular or extracellular fluid. They operate together to regulate the heartbeat. As long as the person does not take diuretics or cortisones, and does not suffer from kidney diseases or diarrhea and vomiting, potassium will be supplied naturally by his diet.

Many of the actions of potassium are performed in conjunction with another mineral, as we stated above. Potassium also works with calcium to regulate the nervous activity of the muscles, and with phosphorus to regulate the brain. Excessive salt in food stemming from the consumption of salty foods or the addition of a lot of salt to food, causes a loss of potassium, resulting in edemas (swellings), irregular heartbeat, and muscle damage. Sometimes, it is also an important factor in high blood pressure; tea, coffee, and alcohol, as well as drastic weight reduction have the same effect.

The functions of potassium include stimulating nervous impulses that activate the muscles to contract and to flex. Moreover, potassium is necessary for growth and for cell metabolism. It regulates the body fluids (together with sodium), and is required for maintaining their alkalinity.

Potassium activates and stimulates the kidneys, and maintains the adrenal glands, which are responsible for fatigue and allergies. Potassium plays an important part in the process of transforming glucose into glycogen. It is connected with conveying oxygen to the brain, and is important for the balance (and lowering) of blood pressure. Finally, potassium is important for the health of the skin.

While there is no daily recommended dietary allowance of potassium, infants up to one year should have 350-1,300 mg, while children over one year should have up to 2,000 mg.

In conditions of stress or sugar problems, or when consuming sugars, the amounts should be increased.

Adults should have 2,000-2,500 mg per day. People who drink coffee, tea, or alcohol should increase the amount, as should those with sugar and blood pressure problems, or those who take diuretics or who are on a carbohydrate-free diet.

Potassium can be found in the following foods: all dried herbs, sunflower seeds, dried onion and garlic, dried fruits, dried legumes, nuts, yams, mushrooms, all vegetables (especially green leafy vegetables), bananas, and all the other vegetables and fruit, cereal plants and fish. It is recommended that people who lack potassium in their bodies, and suffer from tension and cramps in their muscles before jogging or exercise drink a glass of citrus juice in order to get some potassium.

If there is a lack of potassium, the person could suffer from hypoglycemia (a shortage of sugar) that is followed by diarrhea; edemas (accumulation of fluids); constipation and irregularity, or diarrhea; impaired muscle and nerve functioning; various allergies; or tachycardia (abnormally rapid heartbeat).

Similar symptoms can be caused when there is a shortage of magnesium or vitamin B.

Over 25,000 mg of potassium chloride can cause toxicity (this amount is way above the recommended daily amount), so potassium hardly ever causes toxicity.

Selenium

Chemical symbol Se, specific gravity 4.82, atomic weight 78.96 (selenium).

Discovered about 30 years ago, selenium is one of the newer members of the trace element group. It is a non-metallic, chemical element that converts radiation energy (light) into electrical energy easily. This is the origin of its name - selene ("moon" in Greek). For this reason, it is used in the preparation of photo-electric cells. Its action in the body is different.

Selenium retards aging; it is an excellent antioxidant and expels radicals from the body. Thus, it fortifies the immune system and reduces heart attacks.

Research has shown that there is an inverse relation between contracting cancer and selenium, and that cancer patients have been found to have a very low level of selenium in their blood. Moreover, in regions that are poor in selenium (in food), three times more cases of liver diseases, reproductive disorders, and heart diseases (in children, too) have been found than in selenium-rich areas.

Today, because of chemical fertilizers (sprays), the amount of selenium in the earth has decreased or even disappeared altogether. This phenomenon requires the consumption of selenium supplements. Its vegetable sources (which are its main ones) are onions, garlic, and the seeds of whole wheat that was grown in earth that was not fertilized with chemicals and not sprayed - that is, organic.

Selenium is destroyed in industrial food processing.

Selenium prevents and cures various kinds of cancer. It is an anti-oxidant 100 times more powerful than vitamin E.

It is synergistic with vitamin E (that is, it completes and strengthens it) and distributes the vitamin in the body, thus creating antibodies for the immune system. It breaks down and purifies toxic chemical compounds and heavy metals. It prevents lead, cadmium, and mercury poisoning, and gets rid of mercury toxicity. It helps to create hard protein compounds, thus helping hair and nails. It is helpful in maintaining the beauty and elasticity of the skin and the hair, and prevents dandruff. It maintains the normal state of the muscles (including the heart muscle). It is important for the treatment of allergies caused by environmental pollution (in therapeutic doses). It decreases hot flashes and other problems of menopause. It helps to prevent heart diseases.

There is no daily recommended dietary allowance for selenium. The estimated safe daily intake is as follows: for infants of up to 6 months, it is 0.01-0.04 mg, for infants of between 6 and 12 months, it is 0.02-0.06 mg, for children of between 1 and 3 years, it is 0.02-0.08 mg, for children of between 4 and 6 years, it is 0.03-0.12 mg, for children of between 7 and 10 years, it is 0.05-0.20 mg, for people of 11 years and over, it is 0.06-0.20 mg. Children should not be administered therapeutic doses, as selenium is liable to take the place of fluorine.

Selenium is found in the following foods: onions, bean sprouts, tomatoes, broccoli, whole grains and wheat germ (that were not sprayed with chemicals), marine fish and sea food, and brewer's yeast (not torula yeast).

If there is a shortage of selenium, the following symptoms may occur: low resistance to disease; a greater susceptibility to malignant diseases; muscle diseases and muscle weakness throughout the body (including the heart muscle); degenerative liver diseases; general reproductive disorders; atherosclerosis, high blood pressure.

Generally speaking, there is no fear of toxicity because of the lack of selenium in food; having said that, toxicity can result from very high doses that are not part of a supervised treatment. In therapeutic doses, when there is a shortage of selenium in the body (as in the case of cancer), higher therapeutic doses are generally given.

Silicon

Chemical symbol Si, specific gravity 2.33, atomic weight 28.06 (silicium).

Silicon is a non-metallic, chemical element. It is gray in color, and crystalline in structure. It is the main element in the world of rocks and minerals of which the crust of the earth is composed. It occurs naturally as silicate (a salt of silicic acid).

Until recent years, it was thought that since it is the most common element, there is no danger of a shortage, but tests reveal that silicon shortages occur in the body, mainly because of poor nutrition, lacking in minerals (junk food), which leads to symptoms of shortage.

If there is a shortage of silicon, the following symptoms may occur: skin problems; bone weakness; hair problems (mainly hair loss); nail problems (mainly split nails).

No toxicity of silicon has been found, and there are no daily recommended dietary allowances. Silicon is found in plants (such as horse-tail). If there are signs of a lack of silicon, or if tests (such as hair tests) reveal a shortage, silicon must be taken as a supplement for a long time. Experience has shown that a reasonable period of time for seeing positive results (after the absorption of silicon in the body) is between three months and a year.

Sodium

Chemical symbol Na, specific gravity 0.97, atomic weight 23 (natrium).

Sodium is a soft metal, with a silvery color and shine that quickly disappears upon exposure to air because of its tendency to oxidize rapidly.

Sodium is found in the extracellular fluid in our bodies: blood and lymph. In contrast, potassium is found in the intracellular fluid, and the two elements have to work together in a balanced way. Both of them maintain the fluid balance of the body, while sodium together with chlorine maintain the acid-base balance. This is done by means of a regulating mechanism in the body, which works as follows: chlorine is secreted when there is a tendency toward acidity, and sodium is secreted when there is a tendency toward alkalinity.

Since the daily sodium consumption in our modern world is far more than the body's minimum requirements, there is more to say about problems and diseases caused by an excess of sodium than by a lack of it.

Sodium is necessary for normal nerve action, and for maintaining the tension of the taunus muscles, together with potassium. It maintains the acid-base balance in the body, that is, the regulation of acidity. It maintains the body fluids and is necessary for the production of hydrochloride in the stomach. It looks after the blood, and is responsible for keeping the calcium and other minerals in it.

There is no daily recommended dietary allowance for sodium. The estimated safe daily intake is as follows: For infants up to the age of 6 months, it is 0.115-0.35 g, for infants of between 6 and 12 months, it is 0.25-0.75 g, for children of between 1 and 3 years, it is 0.325-0.975 g, for children of between 4 and 6 years, it is 0.45-1.35 g, for children of between 7 and 10 years, it is 0.60-1.80 g, for youngsters of between 11 and 17 years, it is 0.90-2.270 mg, and for people of 18 and over, it is 1.10-3.30 mg.

Something you should know: Sometimes a craving for salt is a result of insufficient adrenal gland function because of a shortage of the hormone that oversees the accumulation of sodium (it controls the salt).

Sodium can be found in the following foods: all vegetables, proteins, eggs, dried brewer's yeast, sesame seeds, legumes, goat's and sheep's milk, whole grains, nuts, white cheeses, dried fruits, and nearly all fruit. It is found in smaller quantities in dairy products such as yogurt, etc. Table salt or cooking salt are pure sodium chloride, and they supply too much sodium. It is preferable to use pure sea salt, as well as root vegetables such as beets and celery (which is used as a "medication" for high blood pressure).

If there is a shortage of sodium, the following symptoms may occur: Impaired digestion of carbohydrates; flatulence; dehydration; an accumulation of acidity in the body, resulting in arthritis, rheumatism, etc.; neuralgia; loss of muscle weight; impaired function of the adrenal glands, leading to problems and difficulties in withstanding pressures.

The symptoms of a shortage of sodium are liable to manifest themselves in people who refrain from using all kind of salt (including sea salt).

Since sodium is a component of salt (NaCl), most

people have an excess of sodium, and that is because the use of salt is widespread.

All processed and ready-made foods contain salt or monosodium glutamate (I highly recommend that you stay away from that substance), and sodium is also found in baking powder, baking soda, and so on.

Excessive sodium turns into caustic soda, which is liable to cause cancer following the stimulation of the tissues.

Because of the body's (and especially the kidneys') attempt to get rid of the excess sodium via the urine, impaired kidney function occurs, as do high blood pressure, edemas, and blurred vision.

Strontium

Chemical symbol Sm, specific gravity 2.60, atomic weight 87.8 (strontium).

Strontium is a metallic element whose properties resemble those of calcium. It is found in the earth and in spring water. Strontium salts are used for fireworks (they produce a red fire).

Nuclear experiments around the world caused the spread of the radioactive substance, strontium-90, and scientists claim that every human being has already absorbed quantities of it.

This dangerous radioactive substance accumulates in bones during the person's lifetime, and operates like X-rays in the body.

Strontium-90 has the following signs of toxicity: anemia and leukemia, bone cancer, and other forms of cancer.

You can protect yourself against toxicity by consuming the following: algin (from seaweed), and seaweed, pectin, which binds to the toxins in the intestines and prevents them from being absorbed, calcium and magnesium, yogurt and other fermented dairy products, vitamin B complex, lecithin, and the anti-oxidant vitamins.

Sulfur

Chemical symbol S, specific gravity 7, atomic weight 32 (sulphur).

Sulfur is a non-metallic element that is light orange in color, solid, brittle and soft, and highly flammable.

Sulfur is widespread in nature, and among other things it is used in pesticides and black gunpowder. Sulfur is also a component of a powerful acid called sulfuric acid, which is used in the petroleum industry, chemical waste, and dyestuffs.

Sulfur is linked to the consumption of protein, so that neglecting protein consumption (such as by not observing the basic law of food combinations) will cause a problem.

Sulfur is called the "beauty mineral" (despite its attendant odor, especially at sulfur spas), and it is therefore very important not to impair its absorption, since it also helps the blood to be more resistant to bacteria and infections. Moreover, it is found in keratin - the protein of the hair and nails, and in insulin.

Sulfur works with vitamin B complex to balance metabolism. In addition, it is important for the health of the hair, skin, and nails. It helps to balance the oxygen requirements and the activity of the brain. It assists the liver in the production of gall, and as a result, in breaking down fats. Sulfur combats bacterial infections, and is a component of amino acids: cystine, cysteine, methionine, and taurine, which are strong anti-oxidants and protect against toxicity. Experiments have shown that cysteine counteracts the toxicity of smoke and cigarette smoke.

Sulfur is also a component of biotin and thiamin (vitamin B_1), which belong to the vitamin B group.

There is no daily recommended dietary allowance for sulfur. However, it is necessary to maintain the level and quality of proteins in the diet, so that sulfur can be absorbed effectively from the food.

Sulfur can be found in dried beans, fish, eggs, nuts (brazil nuts), lean meat, cabbage, Brussels sprouts, garlic, and onions.

If there is a shortage of sulfur, there is a possibility of hair, skin, or nail problems, and an increase in the body's difficulty to recover from toxicity. However, there are no known diseases resulting from a sulfur shortage.

Sulfur is not known to have toxic properties. The consumption of non-organic sulfur should be avoided.

Tin

Chemical symbol Sn, specific gravity 7.3, atomic weight 118.7 (stannum).

This is a white metal, silver in color, which the body requires for growth.

Little is known about the mechanisms at work in this mineral, except that its toxicity is harmful (like that of lead).

Traces of tin as a trace mineral are found both in plants and animals, and nothing is known about shortage or diseases caused by a shortage in the body.

Vanadium

Chemical symbol V, specific gravity 5.6, atomic weight 50.95 (vanadis).

Vanadium is a rare metal, white in color and similar to silver, which is used in the steel industry and for solidifying in the paint industry. This trace mineral is important for the human body, and even though all the body's requirements of this mineral are not yet known, researchers have found that it is linked to coronary heart diseases.

Vanadium is important for normal growth, as well as for the cholesterol in the body.

It is found in marine fish (abundantly), sea food, herrings, and sardines.

Signs of a shortage of vanadium are fairly rare, and are found in coronary heart diseases, growth, and cholesterol.

There is no toxicity in vanadium (unless synthetic vanadium is taken).

Zinc

Chemical symbol Zn, specific gravity 7.1, atomic weight 65.38 (zincum).

Zinc is a chemical element that belongs to the group of heavy metals.

It acts as a "traffic policeman" for the body's processes and enzyme maintenance.

The quantity of zinc in the body is the second highest of all the minerals, and it is of supreme importance, since it participates in the activities of over 70 enzymes in the digestive and metabolic systems.

Zinc is important for the functioning of the prostate gland and testes, and for the immune system; it helps heal wounds, and alleviates pain.

It is important to know that taking an increased quantity of zinc means that copper and vitamin B6 must also be taken, and it must be remembered that when there is a shortage of zinc, the immediate solution lies only in supplements, since it is difficult to compensate for shortages of zinc, or a demand for zinc, by means of food only.

Zinc is important in maintaining the acid-base balance in the body. It is one of the components of insulin - and for this reason, it is important for the body's sugar system. Moreover, it helps to release vitamin A from the liver, in this way benefiting vision. Zinc is essential for protein synthesis, as well as for the absorption and functioning of vitamins (especially from the B group). It is active in the immune system, kills bacteria, and fights cell degeneration, mainly with vitamins A, C, and selenium. For that reason, it is important in treating the mental deterioration that occurs as a result of Alzheimer's disease. It is important for brain activity and in the treatment of schizophrenia.

Zinc is an important component of the prostate gland, and is a component of seminal fluid. It is an important component in the menstrual cycle, in building the ovum, in sterility, and for sexual development in young people. It is important in the link between the hormonal system and the skin, such as acne problems. Zinc is essential for the skin; it is one of its components, and together with vitamins A, C, and E, treats severe skin problems.

Together with vitamins C and D, it is linked to the building of bones as the "cement" that joins calcium, magnesium and phosphorus. A link has been found to the curing of joint inflammation problems (together with other minerals).

Zinc is used to combat body odor, and, together with vitamin B6, serves as a natural deodorant. In addition, there is a link between zinc (+ vitamins B6 and A) and the senses of taste and smell. It helps to lower the cholesterol level.

The recommended daily amounts for infants of up to 6 months is 3 mg, for infants of between 6 and 12 months is 5 mg, for children of up to 10 years is 10 mg, and for people of 11 years and over is 15 mg. Pregnant women should take 20 mg, and nursing women should take 25 mg.

Children and adults with sugar problems or children who take vitamin B6 require more zinc, as do adults with prostate problems or who are undergoing treatment for problems such as impotence, aging (with manganese) and so on.

It should be remembered that zinc should be taken in conjunction with vitamins A, B6, calcium, and phosphorus. The best forms are chealated zinc, zinc gluconate, or zinc sulfate.

The foodstuffs that contain zinc are as follows: wheatgerm, bran, whole-wheat flour (whole-wheat bread), brown rice, sesame seeds, pumpkin seeds, most dried herbs, cashew nuts, nuts, almonds, eggs, legumes, and in smaller quantities in most vegetables.

When there is a shortage of zinc, the following symptoms can occur: prostate problems, especially enlargement of the gland (not a tumor). Many men ignore the fact that they are getting up more frequently at night, or run to the bathroom more often during the day, and this is a sign of prostate problems. Other symptoms are the slow healing of wounds and cuts, arteriosclerosis - hardening of the arteries, susceptibility to infections, increased fatigue and/or a loss of appetite, diabetic problems, white marks or spots on the nails, a loss of sensitivity to the taste and/or smell of food, and skin diseases (sometimes called "chronic").

While there is no toxicity in zinc, children should not take more than the recommended amounts (unless otherwise directed by a physician), because larger doses over time are liable to cause a shortage of copper, which can result in anemia or impaired heart rate/pulse. Adults should also not exceed the recommended amounts (unless otherwise directed by a physician). Remember to take the supplements.

Dan Wolf

Herbal Remedies

Introduction

The healing properties of herbs and plants have been known to man since prehistoric times. Many ancient cultures actually documented their uses. The Bible, in fact, contains numerous references to herbal remedies.

While the image of the "witchdoctor" or medicine man or woman has been held up to ridicule during the industrial and technological age, and the medical establishment tends to frown upon "natural" healing, there is a growing tendency to return to more natural forms of therapy in order to avoid the harmful and sometimes addictive side-effects of chemical and synthetic drugs. Herbal medicine is a leading branch of what is called "alternative medicine," and - in the ideal world - should work hand in hand with conventional medicine to conquer disease.

It is sobering to think that many tragedies involving bleeding to death, insect bites, various injuries, and so on, might have been averted had there been a basic knowledge of herbal remedies.

This book is an introduction to a few of the major herbal remedies - there are many more - so that you can become familiar with their properties, and come to realize that there are many simple ways of treating all kinds of symptoms and ailments without resorting to antibiotics and other drugs, which have so many negative side-effects. The aim of the book is to familiarize you with the endless potential of the herbs and plants that grow all around us, and to whet your appetite for a greater and more profound knowledge of the subject.

Acacia

(also known as acacia gum, Senegal gum, gum arabic, wattle, black catechu, tamarisk, babul, and Egyptian thorn)

The numerous species of the Acacia genus belong to the Leguminosae family, and grow mainly in Africa, Australia, and the Middle East. These evergreen plants are used for medicinal purposes.

Acacia catechu (which grows in Africa) and Acacia pycnantha (which grows in Australia) are rich in tannin, which is used to treat burns because of its fast healing action. Tannin is also effective in treating mouth ulcers and various oral infections by killing bacteria. The herb reduces unusual bleeding and treats chronic diarrhea.

The branches of Acacia senegal exude a kind of gum whose astringent properties were utilized in ancient Egypt for treating gums and reinforcing loose teeth. It was also used as an antiseptic for open wounds.

The various Acacia remedies must be prescribed by a herbalist or a physician in order to avoid the risk of tannic acid poisoning, which can irritate the mucous membranes in the stomach.

In any event, the remedies must not be taken for a protracted length of time.

Acacia must not be taken during pregnancy, or if pregnancy is planned in the near future, or by people who suffer from duodenal or stomach ulcers, colitis, or diverticulosis.

Aconite

(also known as monkshood, blue rocket, wolfsbane, aconis, friar's mantle, Black Sea root, thora)

Aconite (Aconitum napellus) belongs to the Ranunculaceae family, and is a perennial herb that grows in North America, Europe, and southern and central Asia. It is highly poisonous due to its alkaloid content (aconitine and pseudoaconitine), and anything exceeding a minute dose is lethal. There is no cure for aconite poisoning. Its poison is so lethal that it was used on the tips of poison arrows.

Aconite, in minuscule dosages, is reputed to reduce nervous tension and other nerve disorders, temporarily alleviate Parkinson's symptoms, decrease blood pressure, and regulate the heartbeat. However, there is no safe recommended dosage, and it must be avoided, especially during pregnancy, or if pregnancy is planned in the near future, or by people who suffer from duodenal or stomach ulcers, colitis, or diverticulosis.

Angelica

(also known as European angelica, angel root, garden angelica)

Angelica archangelica belongs to the Umbelliferae family, and grows in northern temperate regions. In particular, it flourishes in New Zealand. While it is used as a flavoring in baking, it also has several therapeutic uses - for instance, for digestive problems, when it helps the body to expel stomach and intestinal gas. In addition, it is used for treating bladder infections, as it contains antiseptic properties, and is a mild diuretic, thus flushing out the harmful bacteria. It relieves mucous congestion in the lungs and bronchial tubes.

The recommended dosage of angelica is 25 grains of powdered root. However, it must not be taken during pregnancy, or if pregnancy is planned in the near future, or by people who suffer from duodenal or stomach ulcers, colitis, or diverticulosis.

Anise seed

(also known as include aniseed, star anise, anise cultive, annissamen)

Anise seed (Pimpinella anisum) belongs to the Umbelliferae family, and grows in the Far East, the United States, and Europe. A familiar ingredient in Chinese cuisine and in the production of liqueur, it has been used since ancient times to treat digestive disorders such as stomach cramps. It stimulates the digestive juices in the stomach and intestines, and helps in the process of breaking down fats into fatty acids. It also helps expel gas from the digestive tract. It has diuretic properties, and relieves mucous congestion in the lungs and bronchial tubes.

The recommended dosage for digestive disturbances and colic is one tablespoon of ground anise seed boiled in a half pint of milk, twice a day. For an eyewash, mix a half teaspoon of anise seed with one pint of water. It must not be taken during pregnancy, or if pregnancy is planned in the near future, or by people who suffer from duodenal or stomach ulcers, colitis, or diverticulosis.

Balm of Gilead

(also known as cottonwood, Mecca balsam, balsam poplar, tacamahack)

Balm of Gilead (Populus candicans) thrives in various regions of the Middle East, especially in Mecca (hence one of its names). The buds are taken from this small shrub in order to produce the oils that are absorbed via the skin. It has anti-inflammatory and antibiotic properties, reducing pain and fever, as well as shortening the course of colds and flu when applied in the form of a cream or a lotion to the chest. It can be an ingredient in antitussives. Because of its antiseptic properties, it is effective in treating infected wounds and skin ulcers. It is reputed to relieve toothache, and to treat heart diseases and arthritis.

The recommended dosage is no more than ten grains in 24 hours. It must not be taken during pregnancy, or if pregnancy is planned in the near future.

Belladonna

(also known as deadly nightshade, black cherry root, dwale)

Belladonna (Atropa belladonna) belongs to the Solanaceae family, and grows throughout southern and central Europe, parts of India and Pakistan, and the southern regions of the United Kingdom.

This is a well-known poison (because of the alkaloid hysoscyamine it contains), but was also used cosmetically to dilate the pupils and make the eyes look darker and more seductive in ancient times.

However, belladonna in small quantities does have some therapeutic uses, especially as a sedative for treating hysteria and nervous disorders and reducing fever, as well as preventing involuntary ejaculation.

There is no safe dosage, and belladonna must not be taken without professional supervision.

Bilberry

(also known as hurtleberry, whortleberry, huckleberry)

Bilberry (Vaccinium myrtillus) is a small shrub that grows in northern Europe and the United Kingdom. The small purple berries are edible, like blueberries, and can be eaten as is (not excessively, however). Bilberry berries treat diarrhea and bowel inflammations because of their astringent properties. They solidify the feces. Bilberry is sometimes used for treating scurvy, as it is rich in vitamin C, and anemia, because of its high iron content. It decreases the blood sugar level, and has diuretic properties.

Bilberry should not be taken if there is evidence of an allergy to huckleberries or blueberries.

Blue flag

(also known as poison lily, blue lily, poison flag)

Blue flag (Iris versicolor) belongs to the Iridaceae family, and grows throughout the United Kingdom. It has diuretic properties, and stimulates liver function. It alleviates severe constipation, and can purify the blood. It is reputed to relieve arthritis and skin disorders, and stimulate cardiac function.

The daily adult dosage, which should be administered by a qualified practitioner only, is no more than 15 grains. Do not be tempted to use it on your own, as its cathartic action can be violent.

Blue flag must not be taken during pregnancy, or if pregnancy is planned in the near future, or by people who suffer from duodenal or stomach ulcers, colitis, esophageal reflux, or diverticulosis.

Borage

(also known as burrage, borrage)

Borage (Borago offinalis) belongs to the Boraginaceae family that originated in the Mediterranean basin and spread all over Europe. From ancient times, it has been used as a sedative. Mixed with wine, it would raise the level of the adrenaline in the blood. Borage is taken in the form of a tea in order to relieve anxiety and nervous tension, but should not be drunk too frequently - maximum twice a day.

Caraway

(also known as carryways, carrywa, and alcaravea)

Caraway (Carum carvi) belongs to the Umbelliferae family, and grows in northern Africa and throughout Europe. Well-known in cookery, its therapeutic uses have been known for millennia, and include relieving digestive disorders such as feeling bloated, flatulence, and diarrhea; it is effective in expelling gas from the digestive tract. Moreover, it stimulates the appetite, making it particularly valuable in cases of anorexia nervosa.

Caraway is taken in the form of tincture of caraway, or as a tea, which is safe for children and adults. A heaped teaspoon of the seed is steeped in freshly boiled water for 15-20 minutes, and drunk 2-3 times a day.

Caraway must not be taken during pregnancy, or if pregnancy is planned in the near future, or by people who suffer from duodenal or stomach ulcers, colitis, esophageal reflux, or diverticulosis.

Catnip

(also known as catmint, catnep, nep, herb catta)

Catnip (Nepeta cataria) belongs to the Labiatae family, and grows throughout the United Kingdom and in the damper parts of the United States and Europe. It is a minty, aromatic plant that spreads easily.

It is a good antiseptic for treating skin lesions, boils, scabs, and acne, as well as for treating dandruff (in the form of shampoo). It soothes stomach cramps when taken as a mild, aromatic tea, which can also be used to treat colds, fever (it induces sweating), and flu, and soothe restless children. It must not be taken during pregnancy, or if pregnancy is planned in the near future.

Chamomile

(also known as camomile, camomille, double chamomile, sailors' buttons)

Chamomile (Anthemis nobilis) belongs to the Compositae family, and grows in western Europe, particularly in Italy, France, and Belgium. Its main therapeutic use is for treating digestive disturbances; it exerts an anti-inflammatory effect on the mucous membranes in the stomach. In addition, it can be used for relieving premenstrual abdominal cramps.

Chamomile is taken in the form of a tea three times a day.

It must not be taken during pregnancy, or if pregnancy is planned in the near future, or by people who suffer from duodenal or stomach ulcers, colitis, esophageal reflux, or diverticulosis.

Chickweed

(also known as star chickweed, starweed)

Chickweed (Stellaria media) belongs to the Caryophyllaceae family, and grows throughout western Europe and the United Kingdom. It is reputed to be an effective skin tonic - especially if the herb is placed in a hot bath - and soothes sores and itches. Chickweed has diuretic properties, but care must be taken not to impair kidney function by taking too large a dose.

It is taken in the form of a tea, but no more than 8 fluid ounces should be consumed per day.

It must not be taken during pregnancy, or if pregnancy is planned in the near future.

Coltsfoot

(also known as cough herb, coughwort, horse-hoof, foal's foot, fool's foot)

Coltsfoot (Tussilago farfara) belongs to the Compositae family, and grows throughout the United States, Asia, northern Africa, Europe, and the United Kingdom - wherever there is damp, clay soil. It is a hardy plant whose therapeutic uses include treating persistent coughs and bronchial and lung disorders, as well as skin problems. It shrinks tissues and prevents the secretion of fluids. It causes tissues to heal quickly thanks to the astringent properties of the tannins it contains.

For coughs, 1-2 teaspoons of the decoction (a quart of water to an ounce of the herb) should be taken.

It must not be taken during pregnancy, or if pregnancy is planned in the near future.

Dandelion

(also known as puff-ball, blow-ball, swine snout, lion's tooth, taraxacum, sun in the grass, wild endive)

Dandelion (Taraxacum officinalis) belongs to the Compositae family, which grows all over the world, particularly in the United States, central and western Europe, and in the United Kingdom. It has been used since ancient times for cleansing and cooling the liver. However, it is their diuretic properties for which dandelions are well known. Since these properties are absorbed through the skin, especially when children play with the flowers, bed-wetting can occur as a result of the increased urine production - hence its nickname, "wet-the-beds."

A lot of nutrients such as vitamins A, B, and C can be found in dandelion greens.

Dandelion can be taken in the form of a tea, a tincture or a decoction. Two to three cups of tea can be drunk daily. The greens can be eaten as they are.

It must not be taken during pregnancy, or if pregnancy is planned in the near future. Moreover, if you suffer from bile duct blockage, intestinal blockage, or gallbladder inflammation, you must not take dandelion.

Elder

(also known as elderberry, black elder)

The European or common elder (Sambucus nigra) grows in Europe, and the American or sweet elder (Sambucus canadensis) grows in North America. They thrive in temperate or sub-tropical climates.

The stems contain cyanide, and must under no circumstances be used. The roots have a violently purgative affect, and should only be used under professional supervision.

These two species of elder are taken as a tea in order to relieve the symptoms of colds and flu. It can help epilepsy. Some reputed uses are treating arthritis, gout, sore throat, headache, abdominal and menstrual pains, and lowering fevers.

It must not be taken during pregnancy, or if pregnancy is planned in the near future, or by people who suffer from duodenal or stomach ulcers, colitis, esophageal reflux, or diverticulosis.

Eyebright

(also known as eufrasia, augentrost)

Eyebright (Euphrasia officinalis) belongs to the Scrofulariaçeae family, and grows in grasslands and pastures all over Europe. Its flowers are used for medicinal purposes.

The main therapeutic use for eyebright is for all kinds of eye diseases, such as pink eye, sties, and irritations, as well as sinus infections and hay-fever. Its active constituents are resins with anti-inflammatory and antiseptic properties.

It is used in the form of drops or a tea made from the liquid extracted from the flowers.

It must not be taken during pregnancy, or if pregnancy is planned in the near future.

Feverfew

(also known as altamisa, bachelor's buttons, featherfoil, featherfew)

Feverfew (Chrysanthemum parthenium) belongs to the Compositae family, and grows in most parts of Europe. It is very effective for flu and respiratory infections that entail a fever, and for eliminating pains, especially menstrual cramps and migraines. It stimulates uterine contractions. Its sedative properties are good for the relief of nervous tension. If taken in very large doses, it can have side effects, but regular doses are safe. Some of its reputed benefits are treating indigestion and diarrhea, for stimulating appetite, for relieving swelling, and for easing childbirth.

It is taken in the form of a tea, a half cup of which is drunk twice a day.

It must not be taken if you are allergic to pyrethrins, during pregnancy, or if pregnancy is planned in the near future.

Garlic

(also known as garlick, gerlick)

Garlic (Allium sativum) belongs to the Lilaceae family, and grows throughout the Mediterranean region and Asia. Besides being a widely used culinary herb, garlic is blessed with many therapeutic uses, thanks to its vitamin, organic sulfur, and antibiotic content. It also contains a range of minerals: iron, phosphorus, selenium, calcium, and potassium. It is beneficial for the digestive and respiratory systems, is an effective means of getting rid of intestinal parasites, fights bacterial infections, serves as a diuretic, eases bronchial and pulmonary congestion, reduces cholesterol level, and lowers hypertension.

The daily dosage of garlic is 2-4 units of a garlic product, or 2-3 raw or cooked cloves. Nursing mothers should not eat raw garlic.

Ginseng

(also known as man root, finger root, pannag)

Ginseng (Panax quinquefolia) grows throughout the Far East and North America. The ginseng grown in Korea is the best in the world. It seems to be an all-round herbal treatment, with reputed beneficial effects ranging from calming the nerves to treating impotence and diabetes to serving as an aphrodisiac. Research has shown that ginseng, in addition to increasing stamina, also increases the blood supply to the muscles - thus proving itself invaluable to athletes. Moreover, the treatment of anorexia benefits from ginseng. It acts as a tonic, and generally invigorates when the person feels chronic fatigue, lethargy, and depression. It strengthens the digestive powers, thus reinforcing the immune system and effecting hormonal balance.

A good way to relax after a strenuous day is to drink a cup of ginseng tea with honey. The tea can be drunk 2-3 times a day, and is prepared by simmering 1 level teaspoon of ground ginseng in a cup or water. The daily ginseng dosage is 15-20 grains three times a day.

Avoid taking ginseng in cases of hypertension. In combination with caffeine, it is liable to raise blood pressure. Diabetics must coordinate their intake of medication with ginseng, which may cause their blood sugar level to drop. In addition, it must not be taken during pregnancy, or if pregnancy is planned in the near future, or by people who suffer from duodenal or stomach ulcers, colitis, esophageal reflux, or diverticulosis.

Goldenrod

(also known as woundwort, Aaron's rod)

Goldenrod (Solidago virga-aurea) belongs to the Compositae family, and grows in North and South America, with a few species found in Asia and Europe. The plant is beneficial for the digestive tract, and stimulates gastric function. It is a diuretic, thus relieving swelling and flushing out stones in the urinary tract. It strengthens the prostate gland and urinary organs. Some herbalists recommend its use for varicose veins. Research has shown that, despite its high pollen content, it is effective in treating hay-fever and other allergies.

Goldenrod can be made into a tea (a half teaspoon per cup) and drunk 1-3 times a day.

If you have chronic kidney problems, goldenrod must be avoided.

Hops

(also known as hoppe, common hop)

Hops (Humulus lupulus) belongs to the Moraceae family, and is a vine that yields male and female cones or strobiles. These cones contain lupulin resins, which play a role in the production of beer, giving it its bitter flavor. Hops has been used since ancient times for calming down excitability, excessive libido, palpitations, and nervousness. As a sedative taken to alleviate insomnia, it is devoid of all side effects, and ensures restful sleep and easy waking. It soothes the digestion, and increases the milk production of nursing mothers. Drinking hop tea is reputed to be useful in treating dyspepsia.

It must not be taken during pregnancy, or if pregnancy is planned in the near future.

Horehound

(also known as hoarhound, white horehound, marvel, marrubium)

Horehound (Marrubium vulgare) belongs to the Labiatae family, and is indigenous to the Mediterranean region and Eurasia. It is also grown in central and southern Europe, the United Kingdom, and North America. Besides its culinary uses in baking and liqueurs, it is used extensively in treating respiratory ailments. It has antispasmodic and expectorant properties, and eases wheezing, asthma, congestion, fevers, and sore throats. In addition, it expels intestinal gas, and the bitter chemical, marrubin, thins the mucus in the bronchial tubes and lungs, and acts as an appetite stimulant.

It is reputed to regulate the menstrual cycle, to induce periods, and to help expel the placenta after birth - however, it must be administered under very strict professional supervision in the latter case.

It is drunk in the form of an infusion (one teaspoon of the herb to one cup of boiled water), 2-3 times daily. Coughs can be relieved by sucking a horehound pastille.

It must not be taken during pregnancy, or if pregnancy is planned in the near future, or by people who suffer from duodenal or stomach ulcers, colitis, esophageal reflux, or diverticulosis.

Horsetail

(also known as Dutch rushes, field horsetail, Hollander rush grass, bottle brush, pewterwort, bottlebrush, shave grass)

Horsetail (Equisetum arvense) belongs to the Sphenophytina order, and of its 16 species, 11 grow in Britain - mainly in Scotland and the north of England. Their therapeutic uses have not been fully researched, but since the plant contains thiaminase, which is poisonous, it can have toxic effects on animals and humans, causing irreversible liver damage. However, another of its components is silica, which is good for strengthening bones, nails, and hair. In this case, horsetail extracts in the form of capsules should be taken. Horsetail is reputed to help cure arthritis and rheumatism, as well as to serve as a diuretic.

Horsetail should not be taken without the supervision of a qualified practitioner. However, the organic silica can be extracted by decoction (simmering 1-2 tablespoons of the cut and sifted plant per cup of water for 3 hours).

It must not be taken during pregnancy, or if pregnancy is planned in the near future, or by people who suffer from chronic heart or kidney disease.

Houseleek

(also known as Jupiter's eye, stonecrop, common houseleek, Thor's beard)

Houseleek (Sempervivum tectorum) belongs to the Crassulaceae family, and grows wild in North Africa and Asia as well as in European gardens. It is reputed to shrink tissues, and act as a diuretic. However, its main use is as a poultice for all kinds of skin ailments and injuries - burns, cuts, insect bites, acne scars, and so on.

It must not be taken during pregnancy, or if pregnancy is planned in the near future, or by people who suffer from duodenal or stomach ulcers, colitis, esophageal reflux, or diverticulosis.

Juniper

(also known as common juniper, horse savin)

Juniper (Juniperus communis) is an evergreen genus that grows mainly in the northern hemisphere. While there are over 70 species of Juniper, the common juniper is the one that is used for therapeutic purposes. While juniper berries are well known for their role in the production of gin, they also have slightly depressant properties. Juniper was formerly used as a sedative. Nowadays, thanks to their antibiotic and cleansing effects, juniper berries are reputed to act as a diuretic, and are helpful in treating cystitis, gout, and flatulence. They are said to cause spontaneous miscarriage.

An infusion of juniper berries can be prepared (1 teaspoon berries infused in 6 cups of boiled water for 20 minutes), and a half cup drunk several times a day. They also come in capsule or drop form.

It must not be taken during pregnancy, or if pregnancy is planned in the near future, or by people who suffer from existing kidney disease, duodenal or stomach ulcers, colitis, esophageal reflux, or diverticulosis.

Kola

(also known as include gotu cola, kola nut, cola nut, gbanja kola, kolla nut)

Kola (Cola nitida) grows in the African rain-forests, as well as in South America. The biggest producer of kola nuts is Nigeria. The kola tree is cultivated for its seeds or nuts, which are known to have stimulant properties. The nuts contain caffeine, colanin, and theobromine, all of which are stimulants. Although it is safe when taken in small doses, it can only be dispensed with an authorized medical prescription. Everyone knows how hard it is to kick the caffeine habit!

As well as being a stimulant, caffeine is also a diuretic, and its astringent properties make it effective in the treatment of diarrhea. Kola stimulates the heart, but caution must be exercised to ensure that palpitations and irregular heartbeat do not occur. It is reputed to increase the libido.

The maximum daily dosage is 28 grains of the herb in powder form.

It must not be taken during pregnancy, or if pregnancy is planned in the near future, or by people who suffer from duodenal or stomach ulcers, colitis, esophageal reflux, or diverticulosis.

Licorice

(also known as liquorice, licorice root, Spanish licorice root, licorish)

Licorice (Glycyrrhiza glabra) belongs to the Papilionaceae family, and grows in India, Russia, and the Mediterranean region. Its therapeutic uses include the treatment of stomach ulcers, gastritis, and so on, thanks to the combined healing action of two of its glycosides. Furthermore, it decreases spasms of skeletal or smooth muscle. Licorice is also used for sore throats and bronchitis, because of its suppressant and expectorant properties. It reduces inflammation. However, its laxative properties require that it be taken judiciously. If it is taken for protracted periods, licorice may cause potassium depletion and sodium retention.

The dosage is 10-30 grains of the powdered root, or chewing the whole root at will.

It must not be taken during pregnancy, or if pregnancy is planned in the near future, or by people who suffer from heart diseases, diabetes or hypertension, or who take diuretics.

Marshmallow

(also known as bismalva, mallards, kitmi, schloss, malvavisco)

Marshmallow (Althaea officinalis) belongs to the Malvaceae family, and grows throughout Europe, and in the coastal regions of the United Kingdom.

Its therapeutic uses include soothing the skin, and treating coughs, sore throats, and respiratory tract infections (in conjunction with other herbs, such as plantain leaf and calendula flowers).

It is reputed to be a cure for urinary tract inflammations and cystisis, even though it has no antibiotic properties. However, by drinking tea made with marshmallow root, the muscular walls of the bladder relax, thereby expelling many bacteria and clearing up the infection. It is commonly drunk for settling digestive disturbances. It also soothes gastritis and ulcers.

Marshmallow can be taken in the form of a decoction whenever needed, or blended with cool water and steeped for a half-hour - one cup several times daily.

It must not be taken during pregnancy, or if pregnancy is planned in the near future, or by people who suffer from duodenal or stomach ulcers, colitis, esophageal reflux, or diverticulosis.

Mistletoe

(also known as misselto, misseltoe)

Mistletoe (Viscum album) belongs to the Loranthaceae family. The various species are parasites. A controversial herb, there are claims that it is an anti-cancer agent, but this is yet to be proved. It is reputed to be a tonic, a sedative, and an antispasmodic. It stimulates the central nervous system, increases blood pressure, and causes the smooth muscle in the uterus and intestines to contract. It is used for treating hypertension. It is reputed to control excessive post-partum bleeding.

This plant must only be taken under strict professional supervision, as it contains viscotoxins.

It must not be taken during pregnancy, or if pregnancy is planned in the near future, or by people who suffer from duodenal or stomach ulcers, colitis, esophageal reflux, or diverticulosis.

Parsley

(also known as fairy feathers)

Parsley (Petroselinum crispum) is an aromatic herb that belongs to the Umbelliferae family, and grows in most subtropical countries. Because it is rich in nutrients (vitamins A and C, iron, calcium, phosphorus, and potassium), it has many therapeutic uses, such as for treating nephritis, which requires minerals, and several forms of arthritis. It helps digestion. Its seeds are a potent diuretic, thus helping lower high blood pressure and relieving water retention. In addition, it is good for the urinary tract and the female reproductive system, regulating menstrual periods, among other things. It is reputed to alleviate period pains, bring about spontaneous abortion, and help dyspepsia.

Parsley can be taken in the form of a tea made by steeping 1 teaspoon cut and sifted roots or a half teaspoon of the fruits per cup of water for a quarter of an hour. A half cup is drunk twice or three times a day.

It must not be taken during pregnancy, or if pregnancy is planned in the near future, or by people who suffer from duodenal or stomach ulcers, colitis, esophageal reflux, or diverticulosis.

Passion flower

(also known as crown of thorns, maypop, granadilla)

Passion flower (Passiflora incarnata) belongs to the Passiflorae family, and grows in South America, South Africa, Hawaii, Australia, and New Zealand. Its exotic-tasting fruit is very popular. Its name derives from the Passion of Christ rather than anything to do with sexual passion, so it is not an aphrodisiac. It is used therapeutically as a sedative, in tablet form, for cases of insomnia and anxiety, hypertension, and PMS. Moreover, it is an effective pain-killer in cases of migraine and neuralgia.

The fruit can be eaten at will, or 15 drops of extract of passiflora can be taken.

It must not be taken during pregnancy, or if pregnancy is planned in the near future.

Peach

(also known as petch, persica)

Peach (Prunus persica) grows not only in its native China, but in Africa, Australia, the Mediterranean region, and the Americas. Since the Middle Ages, pertussis (whooping cough) has been treated with it. Oil of peach is a sedative, and is used therapeutically as a tranquillizer, reducing nervous tension and stress. Peach bark can serve as a diuretic that must be used with caution. In addition, peach bark, in conjunction with other herbs, such as bloodroot, serves as an expectorant. Peach is known to irritate and stimulate the gastrointestinal tract.

The fruit can be eaten at will, but do not to leave the pit in your mouth, or chew it, as it contains cyanide.

It must not be taken during pregnancy, or if pregnancy is planned in the near future, or by people who suffer from duodenal or stomach ulcers, colitis, esophageal reflux, or diverticulosis.

Pennyroyal

(also known as European pennyroyal, pudding grass)

Pennyroyal (Mentha pulegium) is a relatively unknown species of mint that grows all over the United Kingdom. It stimulates uterine contractions, so its reputed therapeutic uses include inducing menstruation and thus treating amenorrhea. It must not be used during pregnancy, as it is liable to cause a spontaneous abortion. This herb must be used with great caution, as even small doses of its essential oil can cause serious liver and kidney damage. So when you apply the oil to the skin as a mosquito repellent, take care to use minute quantities.

It has been suggested for use in cases of vertigo and pertussis.

It is taken in the form of a tea.

It must not be taken during pregnancy, or if pregnancy is planned in the near future.

Peppermint

(also known as American mint, brandy mint, curled mint, lamb mint, pepper mint, balm mint)

Peppermint (Mentha piperita) is a hybrid of Mentha spicata and Mentha aquatica, and contains a large amount of volatile oil - the herbal oil menthol. It is found throughout Britain, and is used therapeutically as a tonic for the digestive system, because of its aromatic property, and by stimulating the gastrointestinal tract. It is reputed to relieve flatulence, nausea, vomiting, heartburn, morning sickness, and irritable bowel syndrome.

It has antispasmodic and antiseptic properties, which make it effective in treating peptic ulcers. It is used for treating gall-bladder and hepatic disturbances. Mixed with sage and boneset, it serves as an antitussive and expectorant, and relieves cold symptoms, fevers, and headaches.

It is taken in the form of an infusion of some of the leaves in a cup of water. Two to three cups can be taken daily.

It must not be taken during pregnancy, or if pregnancy is planned in the near future, or by people who suffer from duodenal or stomach ulcers, colitis, esophageal reflux, or diverticulosis.

Plantain

(also known as ripple grass, ribwort)

Plantain (Plantago major) grows in Africa, Asia, North and South America, Australia, New Zealand, and Europe. Its various properties have been recognized for millennia. It is used for respiratory disorders, as well as for inflammations of the urinary and digestive tracts.

In the form of a poultice, it is an effective antibiotic for treating insect bites, sepsis, wounds, cuts, and burns. The leaves can even be applied directly to the above, and also to oral sores and ulcers, gum diseases, and abscesses. It halts external bleeding.

In addition, plantain has expectorant properties, soothing coughs and lung and bronchial disorders by thinning the amount of mucus in the respiratory passages.

Plantain is taken in the form of a decoction by simmering a half cup of the leaves (dried or fresh) in 2-3 cups of water for about 30 minutes. One to two cups can be drunk several times daily. Alternatively, juice can be extracted from the leaves and added to other fruit or vegetable juices.

Pleurisy root

(also known as tuber root, butterfly weed, wind root, swallow wort, pipple root)

Pleurisy root (Asclepias tuberosa) belongs to the Asclepiadaceae family, and grows all over the Americas. As its name suggests, it is used therapeutically to treat the pulmonary disease, pleurisy, by regulating respiration, reducing fever, and increasing perspiration. It slows down additional pleural inflammation, and its pain-killing properties decrease the pain of the disease. Its respiratory properties include thinning the mucus in the respiratory tract.

It can be taken in the form of a decoction, three times a day.

It must not be taken during pregnancy, or if pregnancy is planned in the near future, or by people who suffer from duodenal or stomach ulcers, colitis, esophageal reflux, or diverticulosis.

Poke root

(also known as poke, pocan, pokeweed, pigeon berry, ink berry, scoke, garget)

Poke root (Phytolacca decandra-americana) is one of about 40 species of the Phytolacca genus, most of which grow in the United States. The raw leaves of most of them are extremely toxic, though some are edible when well cooked. Nevertheless, it must not be eaten. Even handling it can cause skin abrasions. It has alterative properties, that is, it alters the activity of organs, and is reputed to have anti-inflammatory properties, particularly for rheumatism and arthritis. It has been known to treat skin ailments such as ringworm and scabies, and even psoriasis.

Because of the danger of poisoning, poke root must not be taken without professional supervision. Generally speaking, avoid it.

It must not be taken during pregnancy, or if pregnancy is planned in the near future, or by people who suffer from duodenal or stomach ulcers, colitis, esophageal reflux, or diverticulosis.

Prickly ash

(also known as yellowwood, sootberry, toothache tree, false Hercules, false Hercules club)

The genus to which the prickly ash (Zanthoxylum americana) belongs is found in North and South America, Africa, and Asia, and medicinal uses are made mainly of the North American species - Z. americana and Z. clava-herculus, whose properties are similar.

Prickly ash has invigorating and tonic properties in its bark. It induces sweating, and is effective in the treatment of glandular fever. Its berries, which are more easily absorbed, have a similar but more powerful action.

It is taken in the form of a fluid extract of its bark.

It must not be taken during pregnancy, or if pregnancy is planned in the near future, or by people who suffer from duodenal or stomach ulcers, colitis, esophageal reflux, or diverticulosis.

Red clover

(also known as cowgrass, pavine clover)

Red clover (Trifolium pratense) grows in western Europe and Britain. It is reputed to be effective in treating cancer, although this opinion is not shared by the medical establishment. It is also reputed to be an appetite suppressant, and to decrease upper abdominal cramps.

More accepted is the claim that is soothes the bronchial tubes, decreases coughing fits, and can treat pertussis. It causes increased perspiration, and has restorative properties when drunk in the form of a decoction made from its petals.

It must be noted that another species, White or Dutch clover (Trifolium repens), is extremely toxic, as it contains hydrocyanic acid.

It must not be taken during pregnancy, or if pregnancy is planned in the near future.

Rosemary

(also known as Rose Mary)

Rosemary (Rosmarinus officinalis) belongs to a genus of four species, and grows in the Mediterranean basin and in Africa. It is an extremely popular cooking herb, because of its wonderful aroma. Rosemary stimulates the appetite and the flow of digestive juices. It also has diuretic properties. All kinds of painful neurological diseases are treated with rosemary. Arthritic joints can be massaged with rosemary oil, and migraines can be alleviated by using it, too. As it is a good tonic, it is effective for weakness in the cardiovascular or nervous system, and is reputed to induce menstrual periods. As it is a powerful antioxidant, it retards the aging process. It stimulates blood circulation and is recommended for low blood pressure, chronic fatigue, and headaches. It is reputed to expel gas from the intestinal tract.

Rosemary is good for the hair and scalp, preventing dandruff.

Rosemary can be drunk as an infusion (steep one teaspoonful in a cup of water for 20 minutes). Rosemary tea keeps your hair healthy and shiny. A potful of rosemary tea in the bath is refreshing and invigorating. The oil is used externally.

It must not be taken during pregnancy, or if pregnancy is planned in the near future, or by people who suffer from duodenal or stomach ulcers, colitis, esophageal reflux, or diverticulosis.

Rue

(also known as roe, garden rue, ave-grace, German rue, yellow rue, herb grace)

Rue (Ruta graveolens) belongs to the Rutaceae family, and grows in southern Europe. The plant contains, among other things, essential oil, tannins, resins, and bitters. It dilates the blood vessels, thus increasing the blood flow to the organs and muscles. By causing uterine contractions to occur, it is reputed to induce menstruation, which means that it is liable to cause spontaneous abortion if used during pregnancy. It relieves spasm in smooth or skeletal muscle. Using a weak tea made with the herb is an effective eyewash. Rue is reputed to have hemostatic properties, that is, it halts excessive bleeding, especially after childbirth, as well as hallucinogenic properties. Strict control of the doses must be exercised. It is believed to treat hysteria.

Rue must only be taken under professional supervision, because of its abortifacient and hallucinogenic properties. Excessive doses can provoke severe vomiting.

It must not be taken during pregnancy, or if pregnancy is planned in the near future, or by people who suffer from duodenal or stomach ulcers, colitis, esophageal reflux, or diverticulosis.

Sassafras

(also known as saxifrax, gumbo, cinnamon wood, ague tree, mitten tree)

The small, aromatic, three-species Sassafras genus occurs in North America and East Asia. Sassafras albidum is the one that grows in America, and is used in perfumes and food products (not in the United States, where it is banned because it is a potential carcinogen), and its antiseptic oils are used in pharmaceuticals.

Sassafras is used to induce perspiration, thus bringing relief to rheumatic patients who drink it. It has a stimulating property - and a diuretic action - similar to that of caffeine. The decoction can be applied to the skin for treating psoriasis and so on.

It is taken in the form of a decoction, or three drops of oil can be consumed, according to professional instructions.

It must not be taken during pregnancy, or if pregnancy is planned in the near future, or by people who suffer from duodenal or stomach ulcers, colitis, esophageal reflux, or diverticulosis.

Skullcap

(also known as scullcap, mad weed, madderweed, Quaker's hat, Quaker's bonnet)

Skullcap (Scutellaria laterifolia) belongs to the Labitae family whose 300 species are found everywhere in the world. Skullcap grows in the United States, and is known to be the best sedative in the herbal pharmacopoeia. It is successfully used for treating depression and nervous ailments such as insomnia, nervous spasms, irregular heartbeat, muscular tremors, Parkinson's disease, irritability, PMS, nervous tics, and tension headaches. It helps with withdrawal symptoms from tobacco, drugs, or alcohol, and decreases excessive libido.

It has been suggested that skullcap can be used for the treatment of rabies, but there is absolutely no evidence for this.

It has good astringent properties, and is sometimes applied directly to a wound in order to expedite healing.

It is taken in the form of a decoction, a half cup every three hours.

slippery elm

(also known as Red Elm, Elm, Moose Elm, Oohooskah, Ulmenrinde, Ecorce d'Orme)

One of 34 species of elm, slippery elm (Ulmus fulva) grows in the United States, and is by far the most useful of the elms as far as therapeutic applications are concerned. Native Americans have ground the inner bark of the slippery elm for millennia in order to make a drink that is not only nutritious, but also soothes the alimentary canal. It is both anti-inflammatory and astringent. It is an excellent remedy for digestive disturbances.

It is taken in the form of a beverage: First a paste is made from a couple of teaspoons of powdered bark added to a small amount of milk, then hot milk is added, stirred, and a bit of honey added. This coats the intestines and prevents irritation of the mucous membranes.

It must not be taken during pregnancy, or if pregnancy is planned in the near future.

Spearmint

(also known as mackerel herb, lady's garden)

Spearmint (Mentha spicata) belongs to the Mentha family, and is the most widely cultivated of all the species. It is used as a food flavoring, and grows in Europe, Africa, America, Asia, and the United Kingdom. As opposed to its relative, peppermint, spearmint does not contain any menthol, but rather a volatile oil called carvone. It is reputed to be excellent for expelling gas from the intestines, and generally for treating digestive disturbances. It stimulates the muscular action of the gastrointestinal tract.

It has been recommend as a lotion for vaginal inflammations.

It is taken in the form of a decoction.

It must not be taken during pregnancy, or if pregnancy is planned in the near future, or by people who suffer from duodenal or stomach ulcers, colitis, esophageal reflux, or diverticulosis.

Uva ursi

(also known as rockberry, upland cranberry, barberry, mountain box)

Uva ursi (Arctostaphylos uva-ursi) belongs to the Ericaceae family, and of all the species, it possesses the most obvious therapeutic qualities. It grows in the United States, where it is appreciated for its diuretic and astringent properties. Its main use is for treating urinary problems, including bladder or kidney infections. It destroys stones in the kidneys and bladder, and prevents the formation of new ones. It is reputed to decrease an abnormally heavy menstrual flow.

It is taken in the form of a decoction - a glassful four times a day. One tablespoon of the leaves are simmered in 2 cups of water for about 30 minutes until about one cup remains. A half-cup is drunk twice a day.

It must not be taken during pregnancy, or if pregnancy is planned in the near future, or in cases of chronic kidney or digestive disorders, unless prescribed by a qualified practitioner.

Valerian

(also known as garden heliotrope, valeriana, great valerian, tobacco root, setwall)

Valerian (Valeriana officinalis) is a herb that grows in temperate zones, and is cultivated in several European countries (Russia, Germany, Belgium, and Holland) for medicinal purposes. Its use was first documented over a thousand years ago, and to this day is considered an excellent sedative, and a good substitute for various sleeping pills and chemical sedatives.

Its main function is treating nervous disorders, such as tics, phobias, sleeplessness, and tremors. It is reputed to be effective in treating epilepsy and anxiety.

Valerian is a safe herb, non-addictive, and devoid of side-effects. Its use, however, should be supervised by a qualified practitioner. Children can also use it in minimal doses, as prescribed by a practitioner.

It is taken in the form of a decoction. The dosage must be quite strong (one tablespoon of cut and sifted valerian per cup of water, steeped for 30 minutes in a closed pot). One cup is consumed several times a day.

It must not be taken during pregnancy, or if pregnancy is planned in the near future.

Vervain

(also known as European vervaine, verbena, wild hyssop, devil's medicine, bastard balm)

Vervain (Verbena officinalis) belongs to the Verbenaceae family, which originated in America. It is famous for its delicate aroma, and is used in the manufacture of perfume. From ancient times, its ability to destroy stones in the urinary tract has been recognized. It increases perspiration in the case of colds, and clears the nasal passage. It is mildly antidepressant. It stimulates the gastrointestinal tract.

Vervain must not be taken in large doses, as these are toxic. It should be prescribed by a qualified practitioner. However, a small amount of vervain tea can be drunk five times a day.

It must not be taken during pregnancy, or if pregnancy is planned in the near future, or by people who suffer from duodenal or stomach ulcers, colitis, esophageal reflux, or diverticulosis.

Witch hazel

(also known as tobacco wood, snapping hazel, snapping hazelnut, spotted elder, spotted alder, bending elder, striped elder, winter bloom)

Witch hazel (Hamamelis virginiana) grows in Eurasia and North and South America. Its therapeutic uses are based on its refrigerant and antiseptic properties. It contains tannins and essential oils that are good for decreasing skin ailments such as cuts, boils and so on. It shrinks tissues (in the form of liniments, ointments, suppositories, and lotions).

The astringent properties of witch hazel, in the form of a cold compress, are suitable for hemorrhoids and other inflamed delicate tissue. It can be used in the form of an enema for the relief of internal piles. Its active constituent, hamamelin, is used in rectal suppositories.

Witch hazel is used in the form of a distilled extract as a refrigerant lotion for burns. It can be taken internally for hemorrhoids, varicose veins, or diarrhea. In this case, make a decoction by simmering a quarter to a half cup of the bark or dried leaves in water for 20 minutes. Take a half to one cup of tea, twice or three times a day, or apply externally.

It must not be taken during pregnancy, or if pregnancy is planned in the near future, or by people who suffer from duodenal or stomach ulcers, colitis, esophageal reflux, or diverticulosis.

Yellow dock

(also known as sad dock, curled dock)

Yellow dock (Rumex crispus) belongs to the Polygonaceae family, which grows in nearly all the temperate zones. Yellow dock, however, is limited to western Europe and Britain.

Its therapeutic uses include being an antidote for nettle stings by rubbing the leaves over the painful area. It stimulates the gastrointestinal tract.

The root, in the form of a cup of tea made from one teaspoon of powdered root simmered in a cup of water for 20 minutes (one cup, twice or three times a day), can be used internally as a laxative, as well as to maintain regular bowel movements in pregnant women, who tend to suffer from constipation.

It is reputed to be useful in some skin ailments, vaginal yeast infections, cystitis, diarrhea, or gallbladder problems.

It can also be used to destroy intestinal parasites.

The leaves, however, are very toxic, and must under no circumstances be ingested.

It must not be taken during pregnancy, or if pregnancy is planned in the near future, or by people who suffer from duodenal or stomach ulcers, colitis, esophageal reflux, or diverticulosis.

Kevin Hudson

Aromatherapy

Introduction

Aromatherapy is the art of using the essential oils extracted from plants both for healing purposes and for improving quality of life. Essential oils have been used since the dawn of mankind for healing. Some of them, such as myrrh, frankincense, hyssop, and so on, are mentioned in the Bible. They are all antiseptic, without exception, as well as fungicidal, viricidal, and anti-inflammatory. They do not have the side-effects found in synthetic medications; perhaps this accounts for the renewed interest in natural healing.

Essential oils are absorbed into the body through the skin, and reach the circulatory system, thereby affecting the entire body. Their fragrance exerts a great psychological influence: they stimulate or relax, enhance or decrease sexual desire, and so on. They are useful in treating various psychological conditions.

Because of their healing properties, essential oils are very effective in treating a wide variety of skin problems. In combination with relaxing oils, there is a combined mental-physical effect that accelerates healing.

The quality of the oils is extremely important. As it is difficult to determine, the best method is to purchase the oils only from a reliable source.

Essential oils, extracted from plants, contain volatile compounds. These oils are contained in minute amounts in the plant cells, and their function is to protect the cells from diseases and pests, as well as to attract certain insects for the purpose of pollination. Sometimes the oil serves as a natural poison secreted by the roots, in order to prevent other plants from growing too close to it.

Essential oils are produced from different parts of the plants: Flowers, leaves, roots, peel, resin, and so on. They are characterized by their strong odor and their healing properties. The quality of the oil depends on the part of the plant from which it was produced. For instance, angelica oil that is produced from the root of the plant is of much higher quality than that which comes from its seeds.

Essential oils are not water-soluble, but dissolve well in alcohol, and blend easily with macerated oils, fats, and wax.

By immersion in oil - the most ancient method. Plant parts are immersed in a stable oil, such as almond oil, at a relatively high temperature, for a few days to a few weeks. The plant remnants are strained off, and the oil is ready for use. The essential oil produced by this method is not absolutely pure, but rather a mixture of essential oil and macerated oil.

By squeezing - a very common method, used for extracting oil from citrus peel. The peel undergoes a process of pressing or mashing and squeezing by centrifuge.

By distillation - the most common method. This involves condensation apparatus, by means of which water is boiled, and the steam passes through a pipe and reaches a container with the plant parts, causing the oil from the plants to evaporate. A mixture of plant and water steam passes through a cooling pipe, condenses, and drips down into another container. Because of the difference in specific gravity, the water, which is heavier, sinks to the bottom, while the oil floats (except for clove and benzoin oil, which sink to the bottom.)

By enfleurage - the most delicate and expensive method. A glass slab in a wooden frame is covered with oil, upon which a layer of fresh flowers is sprinkled. A day later, all the oil in the flowers is absorbed into the oil layer, and they are replaced by a fresh layer of flowers. This procedure is repeated for over two months until the oil is saturated with essential oil. The fat which is saturated with essential oil is called "pomade." The next stage is dissolving the essential oil in alcohol by shaking the frame constantly. The fat, however, does not dissolve. Then the alcohol is evaporated, and the pure, essential oil remains.

By dissolving in a solvent - a modern method whose aim is to produce as much oil as possible within a short time. The plants are placed in a container with a solvent such as acetone, xylene, etc. The mixture is heated, and the essential oil dissolves in the solvent together with the plant's natural wax. The plant remnants are strained off, the solvent is evaporated, leaving a thick, dark paste called "concrete," which is mixed with alcohol and refrigerated. The essential oil dissolves in the alcohol, while the wax remains as a residue. The solution is strained, the alcohol is evaporated, and the essential oil remains.

By massage - Massaging the body is soothing and relaxing; it stimulates the circulatory system, and creates an overall good feeling. Add essential oils to this, and the advantages are even greater. The proportion of vegetable oil to essential oil is 97.5:2.5%, or to every 2 ml of vegetable oil, one drop of essential oil is added.

Bath - This is also relaxing, and a good way of making the most of the essential oils, as they are not water-soluble, and they float on the surface of the water. In order to spread the oil evenly throughout the bath-water, one of the following methods can be used: (i) Place one heaped tablespoon of bath salts, epsom salts or cooking salt and 5 drops of essential oil in half a glass of lukewarm water, and add to the bath. (ii) While filling the bath, pour one tablespoon of shampoo or liquid soap and 5 drops of essential oil into the water. This method can also be used for shampooing the hair. (iii) While filling the bath, add three tablespoons of honey and 5 drops of essential oil to the water. (The honey itself is nourishing for the skin.)

Essential oil burner - The upper part of the burner looks like a small bowl. A little water is poured into it, and 10-12 drops of essential oil added to it. (The amount of oil depends on the size of the room). The lower part of the burner contains a candle, which heats the water, causing the essential oil to evaporate and spread throughout the room. This method is very effective when someone has a contagious disease. The essential oil disinfects the air and prevents the spread of the infection. The method is also popular for creating a particular atmosphere.

Inhalation - This method is effective in cases of colds, sore throats, and so on, but must not be used by people who suffer from asthma. A quart of hot water is poured into a wide bowl, 5 drops of essential oil are added, the head and bowl are covered with a towel, and the steam is inhaled for a few minutes.

Because essential oils are highly concentrated, certain precautions must be taken when using them.

They must never be swallowed! As they are absorbed efficiently by the skin, they are for external use only.

Essential oils must be stored out of the reach of children.

Essential oils must not be used undiluted on the body (unless indicated in the book). When used for a massage, they must be diluted in vegetable oil.

Before using an essential oil, it is necessary to know its properties and if its use is prohibited in any way (for instance, by pregnant women, children, etc.)

Essential oils must be stored in dark-colored, well-sealed glass (not plastic) bottles, in order to prevent the penetration of light and air. They should not be exposed to extremes of temperature, and should be stored in a cool, dark place, such as a refrigerator or a closet.

Under the correct storage conditions, most essential oils are effective for three years.

Note: The storage conditions for vegetable oils are the same as for essential oils. However, before they are mixed with essential oils, they can be stored in well-sealed plastic bottles in a closet. When mixed, they must be stored in dark glass bottles.

When mixing them with essential oils, make small amounts only. It is a good idea to add vitamin E in the form of wheat-germ oil, in order to delay oxidation. Add 5% of the total amount.

Angelica

Angelica is a powerful disinfectant, and speeds up the healing of cuts and sores. In addition, it has viricidal, calming, and warming properties.

It is used for treating respiratory tract problems such as colds and flu, for healing cuts and sores, and for muscle pains and arthritis.

Warning: The body must not be exposed to sunlight within 12 hours of treatment with angelica. It must not be used during pregnancy.

Anise

Trans-anethole, which is the main component of anise, has an influence on the body that resembles that of estrogen.

Anise is used mainly for treating amenorrhea (absence of menstrual periods) or PMS, as a result of its similarity to estrogen.

It blends well with coriander, lemon, and peppermint.

Warning: Anise oil has a high level of toxicity. It must not be used during pregnancy. Only people who have a great deal of knowledge of and experience in aromatherapy should use it.

Basil

Basil has disinfectant, energizing, and warming properties. It accelerates the healing of wounds.

It is used for treating respiratory tract problems such as colds, flu, and bronchitis, headaches, stings, and muscle pains.

Basil blends well with bergamot and other citrus oils, frankincense, and geranium.

Warning: Basil must not be used during pregnancy.

Benzoin

Benzoin has relaxing, warming, and expectorant properties. In addition, it speeds up the recovery of skin problems.

It is used for treating arthritis, tension and anxiety, and skin problems such as cracked skin, dry skin, irritated skin, aging skin, dermatitis, and psoriasis.

Bergamot

Bergamot has stimulating and disinfectant properties.

It is used for treating greasy skin, sores and bruises, oral herpes, psoriasis, eczema, and acne.

It blends well with most essential oils, especially with geranium, coriander, lavender, vetiver, and ylang-ylang.

Warning: It is absolutely imperative that the body not be exposed to sunlight within 12 hours of treatment with bergamot. Bergapten, which is one of the components of bergamot, is phototoxic, that is, it becomes toxic when exposed to the sun, and is liable to cause pigmentation spots.

However, bergapten-free bergamot oil is available, and it is safer for use. There is no need to wait before exposure to the sun after applying it.

Birch

Birch has anti-inflammatory, antiseptic, diuretic, fungicidal, and anesthetic properties.

It is used for treating muscle pains and arthritis.

Warning: Birch oil has a high level of toxicity. Only people who have a great deal of knowledge of and experience in aromatherapy should use it.

Black pepper

Black pepper has anesthetic, antispasmodic, stimulating, and warming properties.

It is used for treating muscle pains and spasms, arthritis, and cellulite.

Black pepper blends well with frankincense, sandalwood, ginger, rose, vetiver, and citrus oils.

Warning: Black pepper must not be used during pregnancy. Because of its pungency, it should not be used on the face.

Cajeput

Cajeput has fungicidal, viricidal, antispasmodic, stimulating, and warming properties. In addition, it is a powerful disinfectant.

It is used for treating respiratory tract problems such as colds, bronchitis, sinusitis, and asthma, as well as acne, psoriasis, sores, arthritis, and stings.

Cajeput blends well with juniper, hyssop, patchouli, and vetiver.

Camphor

Camphor has stimulating and antispasmodic properties. In addition, it is a powerful antiseptic.

It is used for treating muscle pains, arthritis, acne, greasy skin, burns, sores, and bruises.

Camphor blends well with frankincense, cedarwood, cypress, and clary sage.

Warning: Camphor oil has a high level of toxicity. Asthma sufferers and pregnant women are forbidden to use it. Do not perform a general body massage with this oil.

The author's personal recommendation is not to use this oil at all.

Caraway

Caraway has antiseptic, antispasmodic, stimulating, and warming properties.

It is used for treating muscle pains, arthritis, greasy skin, and acne.

Caraway blends well with peppermint, fennel, cinnamon, cardamom, and ginger.

Warning: Caraway may cause irritation in sensitive skin. It must not be used during pregnancy.

Cardamom

Cardamom has stimulating, antispasmodic, diuretic, warming, and aphrodisiac properties.

It is used for treating muscle pains, fatigue, water retention, headaches, frigidity, and digestive problems such as flatulence and diarrhea.

Cardamom blends well with geranium, frankincense, juniper, myrtle, and citrus oils.

Warning: Cardamom oil may irritate sensitive skin.

Carrot seed

Carrot seed speeds up the healing of sores and burns, and enhances sun-tanning.

It is used for treating burns, wrinkles, and aging skin.

Comment: From carrot seed, only essential oil is produced. In recent years, various weird and wonderful "carrot oils" have become common. In general, they are produced by means of the following process: Carrot powder (dried, ground carrot) is added to distilled sesame oil, which combines with the oil-soluble components in the powder (beta carotene, for example - this is the substance that gives carrot its orange color). Afterward, the powder residue is removed by straining. This is not to say that the oil is ineffective, but the name "carrot oil" in this case is pretentious and misleading.

Cedarwood

Cedarwood has antiseptic, fungicidal, stimulant, and expectorant properties.

It is used for treating hair problems such as dandruff, hair loss, and scalp diseases, as well as greasy skin, acne, eczema, tension, and anxiety.

Cedarwood blends well with bergamot, clary sage, cypress, juniper, neroli, rose, rosemary, and ylang-ylang.

Celery

Celery has stimulating, diuretic, aphrodisiac, anti-inflammatory, and anesthetic properties.

It is used for treating fatigue, arthritis, inflamed skin, and cellulite.

Celery blends well with angelica, palmarosa, basil, and citrus oils.

Chamomile

Chamomile has anesthetic, antispasmodic, anti-inflammatory, antispastic, and relaxing properties.

It is used for treating tension, anxiety, and depression, fatigue, headaches, migraines, sinusitis, scaly skin, muscle pains, arthritis, acne, irritated skin, burns, cracked, chapped skin, dermatitis, dry skin, oral herpes, inflamed skin, psoriasis, stretch marks, menstrual cramps, sores, and cuts.

Chamomile blends well with citrus oils, geranium, rose, patchouli, and ylang-ylang.

Cinnamon

Cinnamon has stimulating and antispasmodic properties. In addition, it is a powerful disinfectant.

It is used for treating respiratory tract problems such as flu and asthma, muscle pains, arthritis, stings, and lice. It blends well with citrus oils, anise, caraway, clove, and rose.

Warning: Cinnamon oil has a high level of toxicity. It must not be used during pregnancy. As it is liable to burn, it should not be used on the face.

Citronella

Citronella is a stimulating oil that is a powerful disinfectant, and an insect repellent.

It is used for treating muscle pains, arthritis, and stings.

It blends well with citrus oils, myrtle, rosemary, and peppermint.

Clary sage

Clary sage has anti-inflammatory, antispasmodic, viricidal, relaxing, warming, and aphrodisiac properties.

It is used for treating weakness and depression, muscle pains, menstrual cramps, bronchitis, aging skin, dermatitis, oral herpes, cuts, and burns.

Clary sage blends well with citrus oils, jasmine, cedarwood, sandalwood, vetiver, and neroli.

Warning: Clary sage must not be used during pregnancy. Do not use clary sage for several hours after the consumption of alcohol.

Comment: In spite of the above warnings, clary sage is far safer to use than regular sage (Salvia officinalis).

Clove

Clove has antispasmodic, viricidal, stimulating, and warming properties. In addition, it is a powerful antiseptic.

It is used for treating toothache, gum infections, muscle pains, respiratory tract problems such as asthma and bronchitis, as well as lice, sores, and bruises.

Clove blends well with citrus oils, cinnamon, sage, and nutmeg.

Warning: Clove must not be used with babies or young children, or during pregnancy. It should always be used in small doses, as it is liable to cause skin irritations.

Coriander

Coriander has warming, stimulating, and antispasmodic properties.

It is used for treating arthritis and muscle pains.

Coriander blends well with citrus oils, marjoram, cypress, and ginger.

Warning: When coriander oil is used on the face, it must be used in minute quantities, as it is liable to irritate the skin.

Cypress

Coriander has antiseptic, contracting, and expectorant properties.

It is used for acne, greasy skin, bruises, cellulite, arthritis, and varicose veins.

Cypress blends well with juniper, lavender, pine, sandalwood, and myrrh.

Dill

Dill has disinfectant, antispasmodic, and relaxing properties. In addition, it relieves flatulence.

It is used for treating depression, sores, digestive problems such as constipation and flatulence, and respiratory tract problems such as colds and bronchitis.

Dill blends well with citrus oils, geranium, myrtle, and neroli.

Warning: Dill must not be used during pregnancy. It must not be used with babies or young children.

Eucalyptus

Eucalyptus has energizing, viricidal, stimulating, anesthetizing, and expectorant properties.

It is used for treating respiratory tract problems, acne, herpes, sores and bruises, burns, stings, and lice.

Eucalyptus blends well with pine, lavender, peppermint and lemon.

Warning: Do not use eucalyptus oil with infants or young children. (Myrtle oil, which has similar properties, but is milder, can be used with them.)

Fennel

Fennel has antispasmodic, warming, and diuretic properties. In addition, it increases cardiac capacity.

It is used for treating fatigue, gum infections, inflamed joints, muscle pains, animal bites, stings, cellulite, greasy skin, aging skin, shortage of milk during nursing, irregular menstrual periods, digestive problems such as stomach-aches and flatulence, and respiratory tract problems such as bronchitis, runny nose, and flu.

Fennel blends well with geranium, rose, cedarwood, and frankincense.

Warning: Fennel must not be used by pregnant women, people who suffer from epilepsy, or babies and young children.

Frankincense

Frankincense has relaxing, stimulating, and warming properties.

It is used for treating respiratory tract problems such as colds and bronchitis, fatigue, irritated skin, aging skin, stretch marks, sores, bruises, and acne.

Frankincense blends well with most essential oils, especially sandalwood, basil, geranium, and myrrh.

Galbanum

Galbanum has stimulating, anesthetic, antispasmodic, antiflatulent, expectorant, and diuretic properties.

It is used for treating mental stress and tension, respiratory tract problems such as bronchitis and colds, muscle pains, arthritis, inflamed skin, sores, and cuts.

Galbanum blends well with lemon grass, myrrh, palmarosa, ginger, and rose.

Warning: Galbanum must not be used during pregnancy. Furthermore, it is liable to irritate sensitive skin.

Garlic

Garlic has antispasmodic, fungicidal, and viricidal properties. In addition, it is a powerful antiseptic, and destroys parasites and worms in the digestive tract.

It is used for treating muscle spasms, arthritis, respiratory tract problems such as bronchitis and colds, as well as acne, stings, and sores.

Because of its exceptionally strong odor, garlic oil is problematic as far as blending with other oils is concerned.

Warning: Garlic oil must not be used by nursing mothers. Care must be taken when it is applied to the face, as it is very pungent, and is liable to burn.

Geranium

Geranium has disinfectant properties. In addition, it speeds up the dissolving of cellulite, and combats water retention.

It is used for treating sores, burns, sunburn, and arthritis. It is also used in skin conditions such as cracked skin, dermatitis, oral herpes, acne, greasy skin, and dry, sensitive skin.

Geranium blends well with most essential oils, especially with citrus and rose oils.

Ginger

Ginger has warming and stimulating properties. It is also considered to be an aphrodisiac.

It is used for treating respiratory tract infections, arthritis, and muscle pains.

Ginger blends well with myrtle, coriander, patchouli, and vetiver.

Warning: In order to avoid skin inflammations, ginger should be used at a low concentration. It must not be used with infants or small children.

Grapefruit

Grapefruit has stimulating properties; it assists in dissolving cellulite, and eliminating liquids.

It is used for treating accumulated liquids and swelling, cellulite, greasy skin, and acne.

Grapefruit blends well with other citrus oils, geranium, cedarwood, lavender and coriander.

Warning: The body must not be exposed to sunlight within 12 hours of treatment with grapefruit.

Hyssop

Hyssop has antiseptic, antispasmodic and stimulating properties.

It is used for treating respiratory tract problems such as colds and bronchitis, sores and bruises, and dermatitis.

It blends well with citrus oils, lavender, and clary sage.

Warning: Hyssop oil has a high level of toxicity. Pregnant women, children, and people who suffer from epilepsy, or have a high fever, are forbidden to use it. Only people who have a great deal of knowledge of and experience in aromatherapy should use it.

Immortelle

Immortelle has antispasmodic, stimulating, antiseptic, fungicidal, and expectorant properties.

It is used for treating respiratory tract problems such as bronchitis, colds, and sinusitis, as well as skin conditions such as dermatitis, psoriasis, acne, and inflamed skin.

Immortelle blends well with patchouli, yarrow, vetiver, cedarwood, cypress, clary sage, and citrus oils.

Jasmine

Jasmine is considered to be the most effective aphrodisiac of all the essential oils. It has, in addition, antispasmodic, relaxing, and warming properties, and it speeds up the regeneration of the epidermal (skin) cells.

It is used for treating frigidity, anxiety, depression, muscle pains, respiratory tract problems such as colds and asthma, as well as skin conditions, including dry, sensitive skin, irritated skin, dermatitis, and wrinkles.

Jasmine blends well with most essential oils, especially citrus oils, rose, sandalwood, palmarosa, and geranium.

Juniper

Juniper has antiseptic, antibacterial, warming, and stimulating properties. It also releases accumulated liquids.

It is used for treating muscle pains, arthritis, greasy skin, acne, dermatitis, and psoriasis.

Juniper blends well with citrus oils, geranium, lavender, myrrh, and sandalwood.

Warning: Juniper must not be used during pregnancy.

Laurel

Laurel has relaxing, warming, disinfectant, anesthetic, and antispasmodic properties.

It is used for treating respiratory tract problems such as bronchitis and colds, as well as arthritis, muscle pains, scaly skin, and inflamed skin.

Laurel blends well with coriander, ginger, marjoram, cedarwood, rose, and lavender.

Warning: Laurel must not be used during pregnancy.

Lavender

Lavender has antiseptic, relaxing, anesthetic, and antispasmodic properties.

It is used for treating sinusitis, migraine, muscle pains, respiratory tract problems such as asthma and bronchitis. as well as skin problems including aging skin, greasy skin, hypersensitive skin, acne, dermatitis, psoriasis, burns, sores, and stings.

Lavender blends well with most essential oils, especially chamomile, frankincense, and citrus oils.

Comment: There is a range of different-quality lavender oil available. Sometimes lavendine oil (a hybrid of Lavandula vera and Lavandula spica) is sold as lavender oil. Lavendine contains five times more essential oil than lavender, but the quality is lower. For this reason, it is important to purchase lavender oil from a reliable source.

Lemon

Lemon is a powerful antiseptic, and has viricidal, fungicidal, and stimulating properties.

It is used for treating respiratory tract problems (bronchitis, colds), arthritis, cellulite, oral herpes, acne, greasy skin, psoriasis, scaly skin, and stings.

Lemon combines well with most essential oils, especially geranium, chamomile, and neroli.

Warning: The body must not be exposed to sunlight within 12 hours of treatment with lemon.

Lemon grass

Lemon grass has relaxing, disinfectant, bactericidal, and diuretic properties. In addition, it is an effective insect repellent, and stimulates the digestive system.

It is used for treating headaches, inflamed skin, greasy skin, acne, and problems of the digestive system such as flatulence and constipation.

It blends well with citrus oils, geranium, jasmine, and lavender.

Warning: Lemon grass must not be used with babies and young children.

Comment: There is a strain of lemon grass that is called Cymbopogon flexuosus from which the essential oil Indian verbena is produced - quite distinct from real lemon verbena, which is incomparably more expensive.

Lemon verbena

Lemon verbena has fungicidal, antispasmodic, relaxing and refreshing properties. It is a powerful antiseptic.

It is used for treating depression, tension, acne, and stomach-aches resulting from flatulence.

Lemon verbena blends well with citrus oils, palmarosa, jasmine, and basil.

Warning: The body must not be exposed to sunlight within 12 hours of treatment with lemon verbena. It is liable to irritate the skin.

Comment: The global production of lemon verbena is extremely limited, and for this reason it is quite expensive. It is important to purchase it from a reliable source. Ensure that the oil is indeed lemon verbena oil, and not Indian verbena (which in fact is a strain of lemon grass called Cymbopogon flexuosus), or Spanish verbena. There are synthetic imitations of lemon verbena oil available as well.

Lime

Lime has antiseptic, viricidal, fungicidal, and contracting properties.

It is used to treat depression and anxiety, respiratory tract problems such as colds and sinusitis, as well as muscle pains, arthritis, greasy skin, sores, and cuts.

Lime blend well with other citrus oils, lavender, palmarosa, and angelica.

Warning: The body must not be exposed to sunlight within 12 hours of treatment with lime.

Mandarin

Mandarin has viricidal and stimulating properties.

It is used for treating muscle pains, greasy skin, cellulite, and stretch marks.

Mandarin blends well with other citrus oils, geranium, cedarwood, and lavender.

Warning: The body must not be exposed to sunlight within 12 hours of treatment with mandarin.

Marigold

Marigold has relaxing, stimulating, antispasmodic, fungicidal, and bactericidal properties.

It is used for treating hypersensitive skin, acne scars, burns, cuts, dermatitis, impetigo.

Marjoram

Marjoram has warming, antispasmodic, and relaxing properties. Furthermore, it is a libido suppressant.

It is used for tension and anxiety, migraines, arthritis, headaches, menstrual cramps, and respiratory tract problems such as bronchitis and colds.

Marjoram blends well with bergamot, chamomile, lavender, and coriander.

Warning: Marjoram oil must not be used during pregnancy.

Melissa

Melissa has relaxing, cooling, viricidal properties. In addition, it prevents cramps.

It is used for treating insomnia, migraines, depression, muscle pains, respiratory tract problems such as bronchitis and colds, dermatitis, stings, and sensitive, irritated skin.

Melissa blends well with myrtle, geranium, lavender, and citrus oils.

Warning: Melissa oil must not be used during pregnancy.

Comment: In order to produce one kilogram of melissa oil, several tons of the plant are required. As a result, the price of authentic melissa oil is extremely high. The oil is only produced in commercial quantities in France (a few dozen kilograms a year). Most of the oils that are sold globally under the name "melissa" are in fact a mixture of citrus oils that may (or may not) contain a minuscule amount of true melissa oil. Lemon grass oil or citronella oil that is distilled with melissa leaves is also liable to be sold under the name "melissa".

Myrrh

Myrrh has warming, relaxing, disinfectant, and antifungal properties.

It is used for treating respiratory tract problems such as bronchitis and colds, inflammations of the gums, cuts, and skin conditions such as irritated skin, acne, dermatitis, dry skin, aging skin, and wrinkles.

Myrrh blends well with cedarwood, frankincense, patchouli, neroli, sandalwood, vetiver, and rose.

Warning: Myrrh oil must not be used during pregnancy.

Myrtle

Myrtle has antiseptic, contracting, and expectorant properties. It is used for treating respiratory tract problems such as colds, flu, and bronchitis; it is especially recommended for children, since it is relatively mild. Myrtle is also used for treating acne and greasy skin.

Myrtle blends well with lemon, pine, lavender, and peppermint.

Neroli

Neroli has antispasmodic, viricidal, relaxing, aphrodisiac properties. In addition, it accelerates the regeneration of epidermal (skin) cells.

It is used for treating anxiety and depression, frigidity, muscle pains, and skin conditions including acne, hypersensitive skin, irritated skin, dry skin, dermatitis, and aging skin.

Neroli blends well with most essential oils, especially geranium, benzoin, chamomile, frankincense, rose, sandalwood, vetiver, and cedarwood.

Comment: One thousand kilograms of flowers are required for the production of one kilogram of neroli oil, which means that it is very expensive. Authentic neroli oil is not very common, and it is difficult to obtain. Most of the oils that are sold under the name of "neroli" are in fact petitgrain oil that may (or may not) be mixed with a minuscule amount of neroli oil.

Niaouli

Niaouli has anesthetic, fungicidal, viricidal, and stimulating properties. It is also a powerful disinfectant.

It is used for treating respiratory tract problems such as sinusitis, runny nose, colds, and bronchitis, as well as arthritis, acne, burns, stings, dermatitis, and sores.

Niaouli blends well with patchouli, myrtle, lavender and camphor.

Nutmeg

Nutmeg has antiseptic, antispasmodic, stimulating, anesthetic, and aphrodisiac properties.

It is used for treating problems of the digestive system such as flatulence and diarrhea, halitosis (bad breath), menstrual cramps, muscle pains, and arthritis.

Nutmeg blends well with cinnamon, galbanum (resin), citrus oils, and cloves.

Warning: Nutmeg must not be used during pregnancy. It may cause a burning sensation on sensitive skin. It should not be used over a prolonged period of time.

Orange

Orange has antispasmodic, viricidal, calming, and warming properties.

It is used for treating tension, depression, respiratory tract problems such as bronchitis and colds, muscle pains, dry, sensitive skin, acne, aging skin, stretch marks, and dermatitis.

Orange blends well with most essential oils, especially clary sage, coriander, geranium, rose, and vetiver.

Warning: The body must not be exposed to sunlight within 12 hours of treatment with orange.

Oregano

Oregano has relaxing, disinfectant, and analgesic properties. In addition, it accelerates the dissolving of cellulite, and repels lice.

It is used for treating muscle pains, arthritis, respiratory tract problems, cellulite, and lice.

Oregano blends well with bergamot, black pepper, and juniper.

Palmarosa

Palmarosa has antiseptic, fungicidal, and viricidal properties. In addition, it speeds up the regeneration of the epidermal (skin) cells.

It is used for treating acne (and the scars that are left by acne), wrinkles, aging skin, dry, sensitive skin, sores, and bruises.

It blends well with citrus oils, geranium, jasmine, sandalwood, and cedarwood.

Parsley

Parsley has antiseptic, antispasmodic, diuretic, expectorant, and relaxing properties. In addition, it relieves flatulence, and combats water retention.

It is used for treating cellulite, swelling, arthritis, muscle pains, digestive problems (gas), sores, bruises, and spiderweb capillaries.

Parsley blends well with citrus oils, rosemary, lavender, and marjoram.

Warning: Parsley must not be used during pregnancy. It should always be used in small doses.

Patchouli

Patchouli has antibiotic, antifungal, aphro-disiac properties. In addition, it stimulates the regeneration of epidermal (skin) cells.

It is used for treating tension and anxiety, acne, cracked skin, aging skin, dermatitis, scaly skin, greasy skin, wrinkles, oral herpes, impetigo, seborrhea, hair loss, and stretch marks.

Patchouli blends well with citrus oils, ginger, lavender, myrrh, neroli, and rose.

Peppermint

Peppermint has antispasmodic, fungicidal, viricidal, cooling, and stimulating properties. It is also a powerful antiseptic.

It is used for treating muscle pains, headaches, lice, respiratory tract problems such as asthma, bronchitis, and colds, and skin conditions including acne, dermatitis, inflamed skin, and irritated skin.

Peppermint blends well with benzoin, rosemary, basil, and eucalyptus.

Warning: Do not massage peppermint oil into the entire body at once, since this causes a sensation of extreme coldness. For the same reason, peppermint oil should not be used in the bath on its own. It should be blended with other oils.

The oil must not be used at night, as it is a stimulant, and is liable to prevent you from falling asleep. Peppermint oil must not be used during pregnancy, nor must it be used with infants and young children.

Petitgrain

Petitgrain has viricidal, relaxing, and antispasmodic properties.

It is used for treating tension and anxiety, muscle pains, acne, and greasy skin.

Petitgrain blends well with most essential oils, especially geranium, ylang-ylang, rosemary, and vetiver.

Comment: Authentic petitgrain oil is produced from the leaves of the bitter orange tree (Citrus aurantium amara). It can also be produced from the leaves of other citrus fruits such as lemon, mandarin, and so on. In addition, it can be produced from the branches and unripe fruit. The finest oil comes from southern France, where it is produced from the leaves only.

Pine

Pine has strong antiseptic properties. Furthermore, it is an expectorant.

It is used for treating respiratory tract problems, arthritis, muscle pains, and fatigue.

Pine blends well with bergamot and the other citrus oils, cedarwood, cypress, geranium, lavender, and patchouli.

Red thyme

Red thyme has stimulating, antibiotic, and anesthetic properties. In addition, it is an extremely powerful disinfectant.

It is used for treating arthritis, cellulite, infected sores, and lice.

Red thyme blends well with lavender, rosemary, geranium, and cedarwood.

Warning: When using the red strain of thyme, you must be doubly cautious, and use an extremely small dose in order to avoid irritating the skin. Red thyme must not be used by pregnant women, people who suffer from high blood pressure, or babies and young children.

Rose

Rose has relaxing, disinfectant, antibacterial, and aphrodisiac properties.

It is used for treating anxiety, depression, fatigue, frigidity, as well as skin conditions such as aging skin, dry, sensitive skin, dermatitis, irritated skin, and wrinkles.

Rose blends well with most other essential oils, especially chamomile, frankincense, sandalwood, patchouli, vetiver, and jasmine.

Rosemary

Rosemary has stimulating, anesthetic, viricidal, and warming properties. In addition, it is a powerful antiseptic, and a louse repellent.

It is used for treating fatigue (it is effective in improving concentration while studying for exams, etc.), scaly skin, lice, headaches, migraines, sinusitis, muscle pains, greasy skin, sores, and respiratory tract problems such as asthma, bronchitis, and flu.

Rosemary blends well with citrus oils, basil, lavender, and frankincense.

Warning: Rosemary should not be used by pregnant women, by people with high blood pressure, or by people who suffer from epilepsy.

Rosewood

Rosewood has antiseptic, anesthetic, stimulating, and fungicidal properties.

It is used for treating sensitive skin, aging skin, and headaches.

Comment: Rosewood trees are an endangered species because of the unlimited destruction of the Brazilian rainforests. The price of the oil is increasing, and, in parallel, so are the quantities of synthetic rosewood oil that are available. For this reason, you are well advised not to use this oil at all.

Sage

Sage has stimulating, anesthetic, warming, and antispasmodic properties. It is also a powerful antiseptic.

It is used for treating weakness, muscle pains, bronchitis, dermatitis, hair loss, sores, and bruises.

Sage blends well with citrus oils, rosemary, and lavender.

Warning: Sage oil must not be used by pregnant women, epilepsy sufferers, infants or young children.

Sandalwood

Sandalwood has relaxing, aphrodisiac, anti-spasmodic, antiseptic, and expectorant properties.

It is used for treating tension and depression, bronchitis, and flu, as well as skin conditions such as acne, cracked skin, dry skin, aging skin, dermatitis, wrinkles, sun-burn, and scaly skin.

Sandalwood blends well with most essential oils, especially patchouli, myrrh, frankincense, rose, and ylang-ylang.

Comment: Sandalwood oil is produced from mature trees (30-50 years old), but because of the growing demand for this oil over the last years (particularly by perfume manufacturers), there has been an ongoing decimation of the sandalwood forests in India. The price of the oil keeps rising, and young trees are being cut down in order to produce the oil.

Siberian

Siberian fir has antiseptic, relaxing, and expectorant properties.

It is used for treating respiratory tract problems such as bronchitis, colds, asthma, shortness of breath, as well as muscle pains and arthritis.

Siberian fir blends well with myrrh, rosemary, myrtle, eucalyptus, and cinnamon.

Spearmint

Spearmint has disinfectant, anti-inflammatory, and stimulating properties.

It is used for treating respiratory tract problems such as colds and bronchitis, as well as acne and inflamed skin.

Spearmint blends well with myrtle, eucalyptus, rosemary, and lavender.

Warning: Spearmint must not be used during pregnancy.

Sweet thyme

Sweet thyme has antibiotic, disinfectant, and antispasmodic properties.

It is used for treating tension, anxiety, and fatigue, headaches, migraines, respiratory tract problems such as colds, bronchitis, sinusitis, and asthma, arthritis, dermatitis, burns, acne, and irritated, inflamed skin. Sweet thyme blends well with citrus oils, rosemary, and myrtle.

Warning: Sweet thyme must not be used during pregnancy.

Comment: Sweet thyme is the safest oil of the thyme family.

Tangerine

Tangerine has relaxing and antispasmodic properties.

It is used for treating arthritis, muscle pains, cellulite, acne, aging skin, greasy skin, and stretch marks.

Tangerine blends well with other citrus oils, ginger, geranium, and patchouli.

Tea tree

Tea tree has antibiotic, viricidal, and fungicidal properties. It is also an extremely efficient disinfectant.

It is used for respiratory tract problems such as bronchitis, flu, and colds, acne, oral herpes, stings, lice, scars, stretch marks, sun-burn, sores, and cuts.

Tea tree blends well with myrrh, chamomile, pine, eucalyptus, and lemon.

Vetiver

Vetiver has relaxing properties, and is also considered to be an aphrodisiac.

It is used for treating muscle pains, aging skin, acne, and greasy skin.

Vetiver blends well with myrtle, clary sage, frankincense, myrrh, ginger, and rose.

Wintergreen

Wintergreen has antiseptic, stimulating, and diuretic properties.

It is used for treating arthritis, muscle pains, and cellulite.

Warning: Wintergreen oil has a high level of toxicity. Only people who have a great deal of knowledge of and experience in aromatherapy should use it.

Yarrow

Yarrow has anti-inflammatory, antispasmodic, stimulating properties. It speeds up the healing of sores.

It is used for treating sores and cuts, irritated skin, acne, cellulite, spiderweb capillaries, and dermatitis.

Yarrow blends well with myrtle, hyssop, clary sage, and eucalyptus.

Warning: The body must not be exposed to sunlight within 12 hours of treatment with yarrow.

Ylang-ylang

Ylang-ylang has antiseptic, relaxing, and aphrodisiac properties.

It is used for treating greasy skin, mixed skin, and aging skin, and for frigidity.

Ylang-ylang blends well with cedar, patchouli, chamomile, rose, jasmine, and sandalwood.

Susan Holden

Bach Flowers

Introduction

Bach Flower Remedies were devised by a British general practitioner in the first third of the 20th century. Dr. Edward Bach, who was born in 1886, had a large general medical practice. Over the years, he discerned a certain trend among his patients: When they were in some kind of stressful or anxiety-provoking situation, they suffered from a wide range of symptoms. As a responsible and cautious GP, Dr. Bach would carefully treat these symptoms. However, he began to realize that although the patients were gaining a certain amount of symptomatic relief, he was not actually getting to the very root of their problems, which, in general, lay in the psychological realm.

Dr. Bach reached the conclusion that body and mind were an interreacting entity, and that the patient's psychological condition exerted a substantial influence on his physical state: in other words, one aspect could not be treated without relating to the other. If the root of the problem is treated, the ailment will be cured far more effectively than if just the symptoms are treated. Dr. Bach maintained that if symp-tomatic treatment alone was administered, the basic problem would remain, and the disease would never really be eradicated. He decided that the solution to this "body-mind" treatment problem lay in plants. He began to study homeopathy and pharmacology, specializing in flowers, and classifying them according to their effect on the psychological conditions that lay at the root of many illnesses. His first set of extracts was called "The Twelve Healers".

In the 1930s, Dr. Bach devised a set of 38 flower extracts, or remedies divided into seven categories according to the particular emotional disorder for which each one was suitable. He laid down precise ground rules for diagnosing the illnesses, and provided instructions for the production and dosage of the remedies.

Dr. Bach's "rescue package" consisted of five extracts, to be used in emergencies.

Bach Flower Remedies have no negative effects, and can be combined safely. The average dose is 2-4 drops diluted in water, three times a day, or applied directly to the skin.

The extracts are numbered according to the alphabetical order of the names of the flowers.

Bach Flowers

Agrimony

Agrimony is appropriate for people who are prone to deep suffering and severe mental agony, but outwardly continue to smile and conceal their true state. These types can be the very people to whom everyone turns with their troubles, since they always provide a shoulder to cry on. While they are the life and soul of the party, and make everyone laugh, they are in fact in a poor mental or physical condition and need a shoulder or a helping hand. However, they will never reveal this fact to anyone.

This essence is also effective in situations of grief and loss, when the person has not managed to give vent to his pain and let it out, but continues to keep it pent up inside. These people sometimes tend to be afraid of being left alone or of having nothing to do, because they are unable to confront their emotions. They are also often afraid of vocal confrontations and arguments.

Agrimony can cause the person to feel like he's "taking off a mask," by evoking emotions and sometimes torrents of tears. This is a positive reaction, because these emotions needed to be released.

Physical symptoms: Ear and throat infections, sinus problems, chronic hoarseness, thyroid disorders, high blood pressure, and heart problems.

Characteristic sentences:

"Everything's fine, wonderful."

"Don't worry, I always get by."

Aspen

Aspen is used for treating fear or anxiety whose source is unknown. The physiological response to anxiety may be accelerated heartbeat, weakness, spasms, or tremor in the muscles, insomnia, cold sweat, and so forth.

There is probably a reason for the anxiety, but it is not conscious, and the patient is unable to define it. The sensation of fear is liable to appear in the company of other people, without rhyme or reason. When the anxiety is reduced, the patient is able to view his life more clearly, and to understand what is happening to him.

Possible physical symptoms: Cold sweat, weakness in the knees, accelerated heartbeat, rapid breathing, confused thought processes, vertigo, faintness, bladder infections, urinary incontinence, and impotence.

Aspen is a characteristic remedy for difficult periods in life and for periods in which the nervous system is upset or exhausted. It is also used in situations of weakness and muscular tremors resulting from excessive caffeine or (symptomatic) anorexia.

The essence soothes the patient, and when his level of anxiety is reduced, he can look at his life clearly and understand what is happening to him.

Beech

Beech is appropriate for types who are critical and intolerant, and who cannot understand that everyone is born with different talents and chooses a different way of life. They are constantly criticizing people, seeing every flaw and everything that needs correcting (in their opinion), and they don't mince words about it. Nothing is ever "perfect" in their eyes. These types not only repress their emotions, but they are unaware of them; they are therefore incapable of understanding the emotions of others. They can be cynical and harsh to the point of negating the person opposite them. They are inclined to demand more of others than of themselves, and they seem to ignore their own faults. Sometimes they use humor to camouflage their criticism of strangers, but within the family circle, they can be lethal.

Often the source of this imbalance stems from having grown up under a microscope and being constantly criticized as children.

Physical symptoms: Various digestive problems, inflexibility in the skeletal system and the neck, joint problems, back problems, chronic constipation, and a general lack of flow in the body (because of their rigidity of thoughts and emotions, as well as their failure to go with the flow).

Characteristic sentences: "Why can't you be like the neighbors' son?" "How can you be so messy?"

The action of beech causes them to see themselves as they really are, creating a situation of introspection that can sometimes be rather shocking, but very positive.

Centaury

Centaury is for people who are extremely shy, and who go through life in the shadow of stronger and more dominant people without devoting energy to their own development. These people do not know how to say "no" and set limits. They tend to subjugate themselves voluntarily to people who are more forceful than they, and are consequently sometimes taken advantage of. They are inclined to place themselves last in the order of priorities, and allow other people to exploit them.

Centaury is also good for children who are weak and bashful, for premature babies, for states of recuperation after a long illness, when the person feels that he is incapable of making an effort, and for the recovery of the body after strict dieting. The essence can be fortifying for weak muscles or general weakness.

Characteristic sentences: "Don't pay any attention to me," "You don't have to worry about me."

Physical symptoms: Problems with the kidneys because of guilt feelings and fear, impotence, extreme fatigue, respiratory problems, pallor, dark rings under the eyes, stooped posture and a lack of energy, small weak babies, and premature infants.

The essence is known for "breaking bonds," and a person who has been like a browbeaten slave to others all his life can suddenly stand proudly erect.

Cerato

People of this type are drastically lacking in confidence in their knowledge and their decisions. They have a hard time making independent decisions, and tend to accept other people's opinions easily. They are extremely compulsive advice-seekers, hoard information obsessively, and are incapable of deciding what is correct. In spite of their extensive bank of information, they have difficulty applying it because of their lack of confidence in their internal knowledge and their failure to heed their inner voice. They are liable to change their mind time and time again, under the influence of other people's opinions. They can be very dependent, and admire people who take a stand, because of their lack of confidence in their own judgement. They find it difficult to concentrate on their studies because of their lack of confidence in their own knowledge. The result is an inability to decide based on a lack of confidence.

Cerato is also appropriate for any situation in which the person is unable to decide between various things, when he experiences temporary confusion, the feeling of standing at a crossroads without knowing which way to turn, a loss of inner identity, and a lack of confidence in personal knowledge.

Characteristic sentences: "I'm not sure, I don't understand." "I don't know and therefore I am incapable of deciding, or carrying out the task." "What do you think I should do?"

Physical symptoms: Tension headaches, lack of concentration, constant stress.

Cerato helps the person focus, and facilitates decision-making. It helps him know what he really wants.

Cherry plum

Cherry plum is involved with the wholeness of the soul, with sanity, and with the fear of losing control. It is suitable for treating nervous breakdowns, an extreme lack of concentration, the fear of losing control, and the fear of going insane. Often, a Cherry Plum situation is characteristic of hormonal changes. Extreme cases include people who did in fact lose control and were hospitalized in psychiatric wards, and people who had a nervous breakdown because they gave up and could no longer cope with things. Physical symptoms: All the phenomena of loss of control, such as loss of sphincter or bladder control, severe confusion, and anxieties.

Characteristic sentences: "If you don't restrain me, I'll kill him," "If I don't change jobs, I'm going to commit suicide." "I don't have the strength to keep on suffering." "I'm afraid I'll kill myself some day." "I feel like I'm going crazy." "I say and do things, but it isn't really me."

For all those who have lost control, cherry plum pulls them together and centers them. At first, they are liable to lose control even more, in every way possible - more urination, more bowel movements, more crying, losing all sorts of things, not getting up on time in the mornings, and so on. Sometimes this lack of control frightens them enormously because of unanticipated things that occur, for example, unexpected guests suddenly show up - something that has never happened to them. Suddenly they become spontaneous and do things without planning them beforehand. The essence gradually centers them and induces a feeling of spiritual peace, while reducing their fear of losing their sanity. It gets them to see things in the proper perspective.

Chestnut bud

Chestnut bud is a metamorphic essence that causes a return to the past and a move into the future, removing the hurdles so that the person can progress. This essence is characteristic of the type of people for whom the past has no meaning. They experience a lack of progress because they do not learn from the mistakes of the past, and tend to repeat them over and over again. For them, the experiences of the past are erased; each experience is isolated and is not connected to things that have happened before.

This essence constitutes learning - it teaches the person to bridge between the internal state, that is to say, the internal feeling, and the real conditions that prevail in his surroundings. Chestnut bud is also appropriate for people with learning disabilities and with emotional problems created while studying, and helps with memory problems as well.

Characteristic sentences are: "Every boss walks all over me." "Every man hits me." "In every job I get low wages."

Taking the essence is likely to make the person experience things he had long since forgotten - encounters with people from the past, and so on. The moment the experience reemerges, the person is granted an additional opportunity to examine it and learn from it.

Chicory

Chicory helps people who are overly focused on themselves, in addition to being materialistic and full of self-pity. Moreover, they don't know how to give unconditional love. These types are liable to subject others to emotional blackmail, "forcing" people to give them love, and expecting something back in return for everything they give. They can be manipulative, and arouse perpetual guilt feelings in those close to them. For example, they can be overprotective parents in the extreme, smothering their children with love and interfering in their lives incessantly. This situation frequently stems from a loveless childhood that has left the person with an inner vacuum that he is trying to fill by seeking recognition and affection from other people; he has a desperate fear of being abandoned. These types need constant attention, tend to be easily hurt or insulted, and demand respect. They see the world only in relation to themselves: "Whoever treats me nicely is 'good' and whoever does not is 'bad.'" Sometimes they are even capable of creating provocations and behaving in a negative manner, just to attract attention.

Physical symptoms: Stomach problems, problems with the liver and gall bladder, skin ailments, psoriasis, respiratory problems, asthma, bulimia.

Characteristic sentences: "I give you everything and you don't care about me." "Look what I've done for you." "Don't ask me why I'm hurt - you know why!"

Chicory gives a feeling of calmness, quiet, and space. Suddenly the person is able to make the connection between deeds and emotions, and sometimes the need to be alone arises, while the need for constant attention from those around him diminishes. The person feels more loved, and no longer searches for so much love from other people.

Clematis

Clematis is the essence for people who are "spaced out," whose head is in the clouds. Instead of dealing with life, they are immersed in daydreams, living in a fantasy future, and failing to deal with day-to-day life. They may be characterized by apathy, inertia, confusion, and forgetfulness due to lack of attention and fatigue resulting from boredom. There is always someone else who will assume the responsibility, since they cannot be relied on. They usually stick to someone who will do the job for them.

A Clematis type can fall asleep anywhere; adults escape into television and movies, women and girls vicariously live the lives of soap-opera heroes, around whom their entire existence revolves.

Clematis is also appropriate for the following situations: fainting and loss of consciousness; people described as "vegetable" can be treated with it, though it is rubbed on the forehead and temples rather than taken orally; people who engage in meditation and find it difficult to get back to earth; and all situations in which a person feels that he is not being practical. The most extreme case of the essence can be found in autism and in hyperactive children who are unable to concentrate.

The Clematis essence is also good for lack of concentration and attention deficit, and promotes concentration.

Physical symptoms: Slow and unfocused speech, staring eyes, weakness, faintness, a feeling of floating, a lack of stability in the feet, and any situation of being "uprooted" from the ground and reality in an exaggerated way.

This essence grounds a person and helps him become more practical and active in everyday life.

Crab apple

Crab apple is an essence for physical and mental cleansing. It is appropriate for people who feel that they are "dirty" or "impure." In extreme instances, the imbalance can reach the point of compulsive cleanliness ("cleanliness freaks").

This essence is suitable for people who are revolted by bodily secretions and by sexual relations, who are ashamed of their bodies and attribute the negative properties of a lack of cleanness to them, and who consider themselves and their emotions to be ugly and unclean.

The essence can be used after situations that cause a person to feel sensations of disgust, such as opening a blocked sewer, visiting a hospital or any other place that leaves an unpleasant sensation (as though they have been contaminated by non-positive energies), and for purposes of cleansing the body in a state of fast and internal cleansing procedures, after prolonged use of medications, for external skin problems, for states of nasal congestion, mucus, blocked sinuses, for problems of revulsion at having sexual relations, and for cleansing and purifying physical wounds and cuts (both orally and externally - but not as a substitute for antiseptic substances). It is used for all infections of the blood, urine, throat, gums, and ears, as well as for bad breath. It is also used in mixtures for women who have suffered rape and feel polluted.

Physical symptoms: Compulsive hand-washing, revulsion for sheets, bedlinen, and any sort of secretion (birth, menstruation, feces and urine, nursing). Among children, disgust for food and sheets is prominent.

Crab apple can also be applied externally: it is good for burns, eczema, fungal infections, psoriasis, and acne. The essence is also effective as a compress for the skin, and a few drops can also be placed in the bath. Used both externally and internally, it is very good for the treatment of bronchitis, throat infections, asthma, and all infections.

The essence is extremely effective as an aid in kicking habits such as overeating, smoking, alcohol, and so on).

Elm

This is a situational essence, appropriate for strong people who suddenly succumb to exhaustion, depression, and a lack of belief in themselves and in their ability to achieve their goals, people who assume a great deal of responsibility and suddenly become uncertain as to whether they are making the right decisions. The people who live with this type are astounded, as they are used to seeing him functioning at full steam, and making decisions with no hesitation. The person himself will say, out of sheer exhaustion, "I can't think straight," and the decision he makes is liable to be incorrect. This situation is also true of the mother who was always strong and functioned well and has suddenly stopped doing so, strong friends who suddenly break down, and a manager who is facing an important decision and suddenly becomes unsure of his judgement. Fortunately, this is a brief and temporary situation - these people recover quickly and return to their normal behavior.

Elm is also appropriate for moments of crisis in which we feel that we can't meet other people's expectations, and they will be hurt as a result.

Bach said: "Take care of yourself - take a break occasionally and go away on holiday."

Physical symptoms: Severe exhaustion, fatigue, sudden and uncharacteristic dependency.

Gentian

This essence is for people who are pessimistic and depressive, and see only the gloomy side of life. The Gentian type's depression and despair always stem from a known cause. This essence belongs to the pessimistic type of person; it is one of the most negative and energetic masses possible.

His mottoes are: "There is no good without bad." "No pain, no gain." "Life is grim suffering." People of this type live the self-fulfilling prophecy; they beckon the negative energies with statements such as "It's not working," "It's not succeeding," and wherever they are, this is what happens. Gentian helps this type during the treatment of illness as well by encouraging recovery.

Physical symptoms: The most common one is constipation. Gentian can be taken to alleviate it.

This essence helps people to see the "half-full glass," and to form a more optimistic view of the world.

Gorse

Bach described the appearance of Gorse type people thus: "With a pale yellowish cast and black lines under their eyes, they look like people who need some sun in their lives in order to shift the clouds above their heads."

Gorse is a caressing essence in the sense of cleansing the initial troubled atmosphere; it is an essence for people who are pessimistic by nature, people in despair, people who do not believe in others or in their ability to help them. They relate very suspiciously to anyone who tries to help them. They are in a state of deep, silent, internal despair; they do not speak out and express the feeling of "Enough! I can't take anymore." They are not suicidal, but they don't lift a finger to improve their situation. This is because the way they see it, there is nothing more to be done. These types conceal their feelings: "There's no point in talking about how I feel, because it won't help." They continue functioning under their burden of despair, saying to themselves: "I've already given up." Deep sadness can be perceived in them.

Gorse is a wonderful essence for people with terminal diseases who are in despair, and for people who have experienced failure with another essence. It also helps people pull themselves out of despair, both giving them strength and ability, and helping them to learn the lesson that the difficult situation is meant to teach.

Among children, situations such as these are liable to occur - for example, when teachers or parents are on their backs, and they feel that their world has collapsed. "There's nothing that can be done about it. That's what life's all about."

Physical symptoms: All the phenomena that occur in states of depression.

Gorse brings light and hope, and the situation becomes more optimistic. While the problem has not changed, the essence affords the possibility of change.

Heather

Heather is an essence for treating people or conditions that have an enormous need of attention that is expressed in a very blatant manner - so much so that it feels as if people of this type are sucking the energy out of those around them. These types tell their acquaintances their entire life stories, not giving anyone else a chance to get a word in edgewise. They are incapable of understanding that enough is enough. In contrast to the Chicory type, who will be insulted, this type is never hurt, and continues to seek attention even after being rejected. This situation stems from the feeling of being unloved.

Physical symptoms: Obesity, a craving for sweet things, hypochondria, and many ailments that occur in order to attract attention.

Holly

Holly is used for treating people who suffer from negative feelings of hatred, anger, jealousy, rage, and loathing. People of this type do not believe that they are capable of being loved, so they project their negative emotions onto those around them. It is worth taking Holly in any situation in which one becomes extremely irritated.

The Holly type is the embodiment of an emotional storm. It is most definitely an essence of love. These people are liable to embarrass people in public and even enjoy doing so, because of their own bitterness. The lack of balance can also be turned inward rather than outward, and then these people eat themselves up, since many situations and people cause them to experience negative feelings. They waste a lot of energy on anger and hatred.

Holly is also helpful in situations of divorce, in break-ups with a boy/girlfriend involving keen jealousy, or after an argument with someone, when that person's anger is not fading.

Physical symptoms: Children with problems of bedwetting and stuttering; gall bladder and liver problems; compulsive eating; constipation; blockages in the female sexual organs; clenching one's fists; grinding one's teeth.

Honeysuckle

Honeysuckle is appropriate for a situation or a type of person that is stuck in the past. Sometimes the person is not even aware of this fact. His key phrase is "When I was..." This situation sometimes occurs after a severe trauma, separation, or loss of someone close, when people return from abroad but are still there in spirit, and when people cannot stop thinking or talking about the things they could have done and the opportunities they have missed. Sometimes they live in the past and the future simultaneously, and pay no attention to the present.

Physical symptoms: Confusion, drowsiness, daydreaming.

Bach said of them: "All we have to do is to maintain our personality, live our lives, be the captains of our own ships, and everything will be fine."

Honeysuckle is also very good for people with Alzheimer's disease, as it improves their memory.

The essence is also good for any situation of stagnation and when the patient's progress grinds to a halt. The essence helps the person cut loose from the past and get him to appreciate and enjoy the present.

Hornbeam

Hornbeam is an essence for a lack of motivation and the resulting mental and physical fatigue, for a lack of energy and joie de vivre. This essence is meant for people who find it hard to take the first step; they have a hard time in the mornings, or starting the week; it's hard for them to approach the boss and ask for a raise; they find it difficult to ask a girl out on a first date, and so on. For these people, the phrase "have to do" plunges them into despair and immobilizes them. The problem lies in taking the first step, and in their doubt in their ability to do so. After the first step, things work out by themselves.

Characteristic sentences: "I have to hand in a term paper, and just the thought of it is making me sick." "If I had a bit more strength in my legs, I would succeed." "I just can't get up in the morning and look at that paperwork on my desk." "I don't believe I'll be able to do that."

Physical symptoms: Headaches, backaches, pressure in the eyes, earaches, extreme fatigue, all the illnesses that result from the collapse of the immune system, or from ailments that prevent the person from beginning the task. The fatigue dissipates when the person takes an interest in what he is doing.

The essence fortifies the person and enables him to pick himself up and take the necessary step.

Impatiens

Impatiens is an essence for all situations that can be seen as situations of stress. The person lacks patience and tolerance; he feels that things are not moving at his rate; his thought processes work overtime - his head is constantly generating thoughts.

This essence is excellent for hyperactivity. Even when the person is physically calm, his thoughts race, and when he's physically hyperactive, he's calm in his thoughts. The energy surrounding him becomes nervous, and he feels that people around him are not acting or thinking quickly enough. His threshold of stimulation is very low, and he's very liable to have an outburst; his sympathetic system may be working all the time and therefore his stress mechanism is constantly functioning.

These people are sympathetic types (because the primary system at work is the sympathetic system. There may be a problem with acidity in the digestive system because the sympathetic system is working more). This type also needs to be learn to eat properly because his digestive system is also liable to cause overactivity of the sympathetic system.

They will probably suffer from an impaired digestive system. Because the energy is being channeled into stress, they do not breathe properly; their breathing is rapid, and their heart may not withstand the burden, leading to heart attacks. They are liable to suffer from high blood pressure, too.

They have a hard time lying in bed and resting; they burn up energy rapidly, and ultimately they experience extreme fatigue and a sudden drop in energy.

Physical symptoms: Nervous movements, problems with the digestive system, spasmodic pains, headaches, dermatological phenomena related to situations of stress, problems with the thyroid gland and with metabolism (the thyroid gland is associated with stress; a problem with the thyroid gland is only a symptom - generally speaking, the root of the problem resides in stress). Children can be very demanding, and want instant gratification. Women may experience a hormonal imbalance.

Impatiens is good for releasing knotted muscles - four drops an hour apart rubbed into the painful spot.

Larch

Larch is an essence for the most basic lack of confidence. The type is characterized by not doing things so as not to fail. He perceives failure as being the most frightening thing that can happen. When he has no choice, he is liable to do things in a way that will enable him to say later: "I told you not to do it like that." It is very typical of children who fail in school and then say, "I didn't study; if I'd studied, I would have passed." They have potential, but they don't see it. Their lack of confidence paralyzes them; they huddle in a corner and think that their opinion doesn't count, and that they don't have anything to say.

Characteristic sentences: "I can't." "I'm incapable." "I won't succeed." "I can't handle this." "I'm afraid of being in front of an audience." "I'm afraid of the boss."

Larch can also help with situations of stage fright and fear of heights (which can be an expression of the fear of failure). The person may feel inferior to others, and this gets him down.

The essence is also helpful in certain situations, such as before an exam, appearing in front of an audience, or any other situation that can be perceived as a lack of confidence.

Physical symptoms: Weakness (body, muscles, skeleton, knees), voice loss, impotence, impaired virility.

Mimulus

Mimulus is an essence for the treatment of phobias and defined fears: elevators, the dark, dogs, closed places, bacteria, flying, old age, death, giving birth, pressure in day-to-day functioning, and so on.

As a type, these people are characterized as cowards: the fearful child, the cowardly adult, those who find it difficult to cope and are afraid of everything, children who cling to their parents' legs when a dog approaches (not out of hysteria), people who huddle fearfully together in an elevator. They may conceal their fear out of embarrassment.

Mimulus reduces the fear. It is a therapeutic essence and not an immediate one; the treatment works over time. Sometimes, after the fear has disappeared, the real reason for the fear emerges.

Physical symptoms: Similar to those of Aspen, but slightly weaker.

It can be given to babies who are easily startled, to people who experience pressure in the chest as a result of fear, and to people who suffer from impotence stemming from performance anxiety.

Mimulus helps to reduce the fear, and over time completely alleviates it. Along with losing the fear, the person may well understand the root of his fears.

Mustard

Mustard is used for treating severe depression that envelops the person like a black cloud. The person is liable to lose contact with reality and to remain in a state of deep sadness and inability to function. Symptoms such as severe depression, the need to sleep and escape, overeating, closing oneself off, irritability, a tendency to cry, a lack of will to cope, and a feeling of "I'm fed up with it" are liable to occur. The person plunges into depression for no apparent reason, and may well suffer from general gloominess and anxiety attacks.

Mustard should help depressions resulting from a hormonal imbalance (including depression during menstruation or ovulation) and problems with the thyroid gland.

Physical symptoms: Fatigue, exhaustion, heaviness.

This essence works quickly and effectively and helps the person get out of his depression, sometimes in an apparently extreme manner.

Oak

Oak is an essence for people who assume a great deal of responsibility, to the point of a physical and mental breakdown. This essence is appropriate for workaholics - people who go to work even when they're ill, convinced that nobody can manage without them. They take upon themselves tasks that others refuse to do. They see other people as being their responsibility as well. Their credo is that life is responsibility, a quest, an obligation, and theirs is the only way except to do things. They don't complain, because they feel that there isn't anyone else to take the responsibility - so they take it.

Oak people are very responsible - a great rock that can always be leaned on. With them, things are always well organized, and they do not leave work for others. They wear themselves out to the point of complete exhaustion.

People of this type do not usually complain, and will not say that they are unhappy, but they don't hide their troubles, either. They don't know how to rest and take a vacation. These are always the last things on their list of priorities.

Because they do not share responsibility with others, they are likely to reach breaking point - possibly a nervous breakdown.

Physical symptoms: Problems with the shoulders, neck, skeleton, slipped disc, and knees; ulcers and heart attacks. The greater their fatigue, the less their immune system functions, and then they pick up every disease that is going around. It is very common to find that they suffer from allergies.

Their body, which is already incapable of carrying the

load, is liable to manifest the above symptoms in order to make them rest a bit. When Oak is experiencing a physical or emotional crash, it is good to administer Elm, since the essence is likely to "knock" the person into exhaustion that will force him to rest for a while. This reaction is a positive one because if the person does not rest, he can expect physical or mental collapse at a certain point.

Olive

Olive is an essence that helps the person cope with severe fatigue, total exhaustion, caused by the body's and mind's "decision" that there is an urgent need for rest. This situation is likely to arise from a long period of coping with mental or physical suffering, from severe sleep deprivation, and so on. The essence also helps in cases in which the person is recovering from a serious illness and is "addicted" to the feeling of exhaustion. The essence is also helpful for drops in energy level during the day. When one has to carry on functioning - for instance, after the after the midday break when someone tends to fall asleep as a result of physical exhaustion and tiredness, but he has an important meeting - taking three drops of Olive before the meeting will help him cope with the problem.

Olive is good for all cases in which the person wishes to increase his body's vitality, such as during exams, moving house, and so on.

Physical symptoms: A decrease in the functioning of the immune system as a result of fatigue - leading to flu, infections, and so on; also, any other symptom that indicates tiredness and exhaustion.

Olive can be administered in any situation requiring immediate energy; however, because the essence balances the body, if the person is in dire need of rest from a physical or mental point of view, the essence will "knock him out" so that he rests and enables his systems to recover.

Pine

Pine is an essence for guilt. As a type, this is a person who bears a perpetual feeling of guilt, taking the responsibility and blaming himself even for things that have nothing to do with him, to an extreme degree - the type of person who begs forgiveness for every little thing. This condition sometimes appears in children, because they tend to form guilt feelings about all sorts of things that they understand in an unrealistic manner (for instance, if their parents quarrel, they're convinced that it is because of them).

There are parents who manipulate their children by means of guilt ("You're ruining my health"), and severe guilt feelings are formed within the children - these are likely to continue into adulthood. The nature of a guilt feeling is that it requires punishment. If this does not come from without, people may punish themselves, and invite the punishment actively. For instance, "I will eat and stuff myself, and my punishment will be to become fat, disgusting, repulsive, and unpopular." "I will spend my entire salary so that I can't meet my payments, and then the bank will cut off my credit and close my account." "I'll develop diseases that are hard to cure" (such as anorexia).

Physical symptoms: Guilt feelings in the body are

located in the kidneys (pangs of conscience), hence these people may suffer from problems in the urinary tract, cancer of the bladder, prostate problems, problems with the uterus, and various forms of self-punishment. There is also the possibility of digestive problems, because they do not digest things properly.

Pine is good for treating compulsive eaters. It can calm them down, reducing the need for self-flagellation. It is good for children whose parents are in the throes of divorce, when they are being used as a bargaining chip, and feel guilty for having to "choose" one of the parents; for people who work themselves half to death; for people who sacrifice themselves in a relationship, particularly women; for people who do not know how to give and receive in a balanced manner; for problems with having sexual relations based on a feeling of internal guilt, sado-masochism.

Red Chestnut

Red Chestnut is used for treating exaggerated conditions of anxiety and worry about future disasters that may befall the person and those close to him. Sometimes this is manifested outwardly by interference in the life of a loved one (a child, for example) out of fear that something is going to happen to him.

Characteristic sentences: "I rang your office because I wasn't sure if you were involved in the traffic accident they mentioned on the news or not." "You didn't arrive on time, so I thought you'd been hurt in a gang war."

This is a very troublesome energy, which is not only accompanied by very severe negative thoughts, but courts disaster. When a tragedy does happen, people of this type say "You see?" "I told you so." "Now tell me that I don't have to worry - it's a fact; look what happened."

The essence is calming, enabling the person to see the unreality of his fears. Gradually these things stop preoccupying him (he forgets about them), and he shows more confidence and faith in those around him and in life itself.

Rock Rose

Rock Rose is a first-aid essence for treating situations of panic, such as after accidents or receiving bad news. It is also effective after a serious illness. The action of the essence is immediate, and it quickly calms the situation down. It is a good essence for all the side effects of panic, such as the hair rapidly turning white as a result of shock, or losing hair all over the body as a result of terrible fear (not alopecia due to a severe illness or hormonal imbalance). The essence is also good for women in childbirth. The essence neutralizes panic immediately.

Rock Water

Rock Water is an essence for treating people who are hard on themselves, and as a result suffer from a lack of self-esteem. They measure themselves against a very harsh yardstick, and consequently never feel satisfied with themselves. They impose a strict regime of self- discipline, repression, and self-denial on themselves. They aspire to be an example and a role model to others, while inside themselves they yearn to feel joie de vivre, freedom, and spontaneity.

The essence helps them to be less hard on themselves, and almost without noticing it, they let up a bit and allow themselves to be freer.

Scleranthus

Scleranthus helps people in decision-making and is appropriate for situations in which people vacillate between two alternatives and are unable to decide. As a type, these are people who waver, and have a hard time deciding to do something or not, to decide or not to decide. Sometimes, because they are unable to decide, they never begin to act. These types are also liable to be very fickle - to the point of hypocrisy - and prone to extreme mood swings.

Physical symptoms: Problems with balance, a tendency to faint, vertigo, a feeling of instability, insomnia, alternating episodes of constipation and diarrhea, appetite or lack of appetite.

Star of Bethlehem

Star of Bethlehem treats conditions of shock, trauma, collapse after hearing bad news; it is for used for treating traumas and serves as first aid for injuries, fainting spells, traffic accidents and so on, as well as before and after operations.

The essence is layered - it cleanses in a layered fashion, starting with the upper levels and working its way down to the depths. Used over the long term, the essence may raise traumas up into the conscious level in order to give the person a chance to cope with them correctly. The essence also cures infections, and is efficient as a rub for fractures, wounds, and hemorrhages.

Sweet Chestnut

Sweet Chestnut is used for treating conditions of bitterness, melancholy, terrible, deep despair, and tremendous, hopeless agonies of the soul. It is appropriate in moments of crisis when the person feels that there are no solutions to situations in which it seems as though he has been utterly abandoned and isolated, a feeling of no way out, of no more strength, and an incapacity to deal with anything else. The essence cleans up the emotional debris immediately, "lifting" the person and enveloping him.

Vervain

This is an essence for people who direct all their energies toward a given goal or toward extremism and fanaticism about a cause of some kind, to the point of coercing those around them. The type is likely to be characterized by tremendous will power and leadership ability, and he harnesses those around him to the cause that he champions.

In a situation of imbalance, he is likely to go overboard in his missionary zeal to the extent of getting into confrontations. These types expend a great deal of energy without balancing their internal energy, so they burn up a lot of energy and strength. The essence is also appropriate in instances of blind faith in a given thing to the point that the person harms himself for the sake of the "objective."

The essence can be beneficial in bedwetting among older children, protracted diarrhea, and hyperactivity.

Physical symptoms: Irritability, difficulty in falling asleep, weakened immune system, tight muscles, headaches, stiff body.

Vine

Vine is used for treating people who are very domineering and tyrannical toward those around them, and totally lacking in flexibility. They are sometimes violent and abusive toward the people around them. These people only feel strong when they can define the other person as weaker than they, and may even attempt to make that happen. These people do not argue: they lay down the law and make it clear with a look or with violent behavior that their demands must be met. Vine is often appropriate for people in the military and law enforcement who continue doing their job at home as well.

Characteristic sentences: "You will do what I say, right now, and without any argument!" "Forget about 'why' - I said so and that's that!"

This essence is very suitable for adolescence, for children who control the house, and for people who have gained power and status and exploit this fact mercilessly.

Physical symptoms: Constipation, stiffness in the joints, high blood pressure, migraines.

A few drops in coffee or tea each day, and the person will gradually become more gentle and understanding. It works miracles, if one can only convince the person to take the essence. (Some people administer it without the person knowing, which is legitimate in view of the reign of terror that prevails in the home).

Walnut

Walnut is known as the "breaker of bonds." It gets a person out of the rut of a particular way of thinking, removes the evil eye, protects and assists in breaking habits, and is very effective against addictions of all sorts. It is very important for therapists who absorb energies from their patients.

It is good for use in the following situations: For treatment of people who are influenced by a power stronger than themselves such as a personality, ties with the past, memories, habits, against the evil eye, for use during a period of transition (any transitional period in life at any age and situation: teething, toilet training, moving house, separation, and so on), for any situation of breaking an addiction or habit. It helps in situations of remorse and broken-heartedness. It works on three levels: Breaking loose from the past; protection - it gives the person a sense of being enveloped in a transparent protective bubble so that he can examine the situation in an objective manner, without emotional turmoil and without being hurt; and it eases transitions.

It is beneficial for those who are oversensitive and require protection; for people who have a tendency to create symbiotic relationships - with friends, family, workmates, and so forth - which contain a destructive element; for people who need to travel and have a hard time letting go; and for children who cling to their mother.

Physical symptoms: According to the particular case.

Water Violet

Water Violet is used for treating people who withdraw and keep apart from their surroundings, so that they are sometimes considered aloof. Their inner feeling is that they are a cut above other people, and for that reason, they prefer to be by themselves. They have a very strong presence, they are dominant, and other people feel very small beside them. They are independent and deep, but have a hard time expressing and demonstrating emotions; they detest emotional outbursts and shy away from physical contact. It is hard to get them excited. They are not hedonists, nor are they spontaneous. When they are called up on the telephone, they always sound as if they have been disturbed; their answers are curt. They do not have many friends; they are cold, emotionally cool types. It is likely that a situation of this sort results from fear, trauma, and lack of love. It could be that as a child, the person learned very quickly that if he didn't look out for himself, no one else would look out for him. Perhaps he learned that feeling is dangerous and that forming relationships with people means pain. People of this type sometimes had difficult childhood experiences of abandonment or rejection by a parent in their past.

Physical symptoms: Problems with the blood vessels, arteriosclerosis, hemorrhoids, problems with the digestive system, particularly constipation, ulcers, joint inflammations, slipped discs, muscle problems, migraines, dermatological problems (if they don't let it out, it comes out through the skin).

White Chestnut

White Chestnut helps situations in which a person feels that his head is buzzing with thoughts, ranging from a song on the radio that he keeps hearing over and over in his head all day, to bothersome thoughts that preoccupy him. He cannot function properly and does not manage to get to sleep. The essence is good for insomnia that is caused by worrisome thoughts. Sometimes the situation is accompanied by overanxiety. These people sometimes talk to or argue with themselves, and they fail to hear what's going on around them because of the internal din. The essence is also good before meditation, as it calms the flow of thoughts.

Physical symptoms: Headaches, earaches, ringing in the ears, migraines, problems with the shoulders and neck, which are usually knotted up.

Characteristic sentences: "I hear my thoughts inside my head" - as though they hear the wheels turning inside their head.

Wild Oat

Wild Oat is appropriate for talented, ambitious, and multifaceted types who are not able to decide what to do with their lives because of their inability to focus on a limited number of areas only. These people are liable to move from profession to profession, learn numerous things superficially, and experience constant frustration and dissatisfaction.

The essence also improves the ability to concentrate and make decisions. It helps the person find his vocation and his path in life, and to stay there, without wandering off in too many directions.

Wild Rose

Wild Rose is an essence for treating conditions of apathy, indifference, being in a rut, and fear of change and the processes of change. It is suitable for people who refuse to accept the fact that they themselves created the situation and that they are the ones who are allowing it to deteriorate; for people who have become apathetic following great suffering; for people who live an unenjoyable routine, but don't have the strength to get up and change it.

Characteristic sentences: "I have to learn to live with this." "That's how it is in life." "It's a hereditary disease; there's nothing that can be done."

Willow

Willow is an essence for treating people who are bitter, who are constantly whining, who feel that everyone owes them because they are unfortunate and deprived. They do not know how to feel gratitude, but nurture feelings of deprivation and bitterness, and complain incessantly. They perceive themselves as victims, becoming bitter, resentful, and depressed. Because of these traits, people tend to avoid them, and they don't understand that they are the ones who are creating this situation.

Characteristic sentences: "I don't deserve this." "It isn't fair." "I always get gypped."

Rescue Remedy

This is a first-aid remedy for every situation - immediately following a trauma, a traffic accident, receiving bad news, or the like. It is also effective in any situation of nervousness, such as before an exam, test, or important meeting where the person feels that he's quaking with fear. It is good in any situation of temporary emotional upset, fright, anxiety, collapse, panic, shock, irritability, hysteria, violent outbursts, severe confusion, faintness, and loss of consciousness. The remedy consists of five Bach Flower essences: Star of Bethlehem, Clematis, Cherry Plum, Impatiens, and Rock Rose. It works quickly and effectively, and it should always be kept on hand.

BOOKS OF RELATED INTEREST

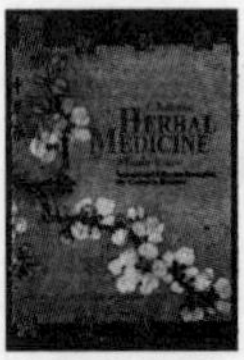

CHINESE HERBAL MEDICINE MADE EASY
Natural and Effective Remedies for Common Illnesses
Thomas Richard Joiner
ISBN: 81-7822-102-0

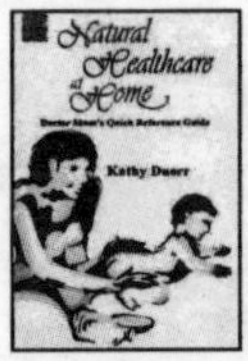

NATURAL HEALTHCARE AT HOME
Doctor Mum's Quick Reference Guide
Kathy Duerr
ISBN: 81-7822-017-2

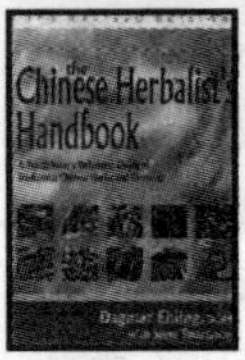

THE CHINESE HERBALIST'S HANDBOOK
A Practitioner's Reference Guide to Traditional Chinese Herbs and Formulas
Dagmar Ehling, Dom
ISBN: 81-7822-196-9

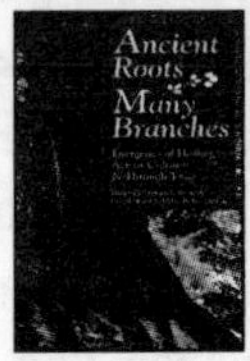

ANCIENT ROOTS, MANY BRANCHES
Energetics of Healing Across Cultures and Through Time
Darlena L'orange & Gary Dolowich
ISBN: 81-7822-126-8

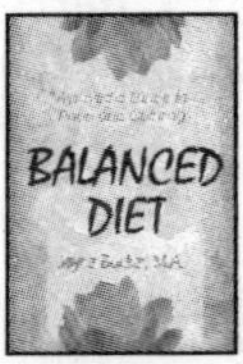

BALANCED DIET
Ayurvedic Guide to Food and Cooking
Joyce Bueker
ISBN: 81-7822-110-1

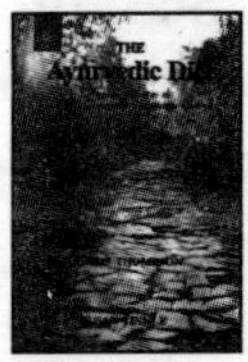

THE AYURVEDIC DIET
The Ancient Way to Health Rejuvenation and Weight Control
Dennis Thompson
ISBN: 81-7822-014-8

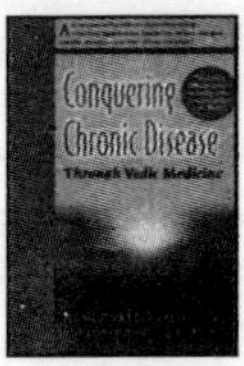

CONQUERING CHRONIC DISEASE THROUGH VEDIC MEDICINE
Kumuda Reddy, Linda Egenes
ISBN: 81-7822-169-1

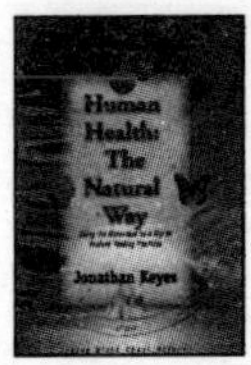

HUMAN HEALTH: THE NATURAL WAY
Using the Horoscope as a key to Ancient Healing Practices
Jonathan Keyes
ISBN: 81-7822-163-2

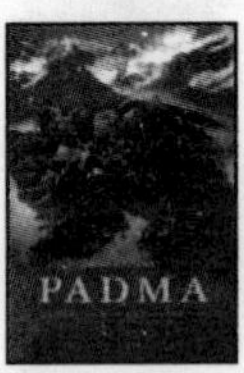

PADMA
The Jewel of Tibetan Remedies
G. Feyerer
ISBN: 81-7822-220-5

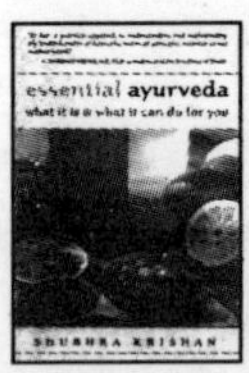

ESSENTIAL AYURVEDA
What it is & what it Can Do for You
Shubhra Krishan
ISBN: 81-7822-216-7

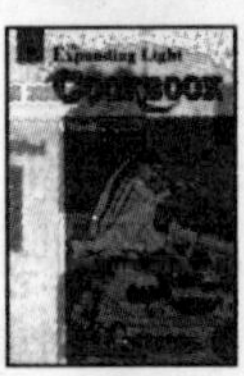

THE EXPANDING LIGHT COOKBOOK
Vegetarian Favorites
Blanche Agassy McCord
ISBN: 81-7822-052-0

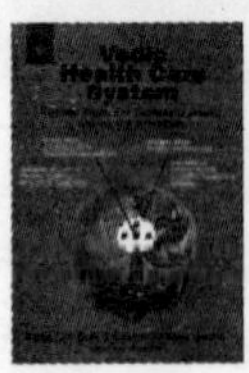

VEDIC HEALTH CARE SYSTEM
Ram Lal Sah, Binod Kumar Joshi & Geeta Joshi
ISBN: 81-7822-041-5